T0235974

Lecture Notes in Computer Science   10557

Commenced Publication in 1973
Founding and Former Series Editors:
Gerhard Goos, Juris Hartmanis, and Jan van Leeuwen

Editorial Board

David Hutchison
    Lancaster University, Lancaster, UK
Takeo Kanade
    Carnegie Mellon University, Pittsburgh, PA, USA
Josef Kittler
    University of Surrey, Guildford, UK
Jon M. Kleinberg
    Cornell University, Ithaca, NY, USA
Friedemann Mattern
    ETH Zurich, Zurich, Switzerland
John C. Mitchell
    Stanford University, Stanford, CA, USA
Moni Naor
    Weizmann Institute of Science, Rehovot, Israel
C. Pandu Rangan
    Indian Institute of Technology, Madras, India
Bernhard Steffen
    TU Dortmund University, Dortmund, Germany
Demetri Terzopoulos
    University of California, Los Angeles, CA, USA
Doug Tygar
    University of California, Berkeley, CA, USA
Gerhard Weikum
    Max Planck Institute for Informatics, Saarbrücken, Germany

More information about this series at http://www.springer.com/series/7412

Sotirios A. Tsaftaris · Ali Gooya
Alejandro F. Frangi · Jerry L. Prince (Eds.)

Simulation and Synthesis in Medical Imaging

Second International Workshop, SASHIMI 2017
Held in Conjunction with MICCAI 2017
Québec City, QC, Canada, September 10, 2017
Proceedings

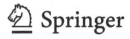

Springer

Editors
Sotirios A. Tsaftaris 🄳
University of Edinburgh
Edinburgh
UK

Alejandro F. Frangi 🄳
University of Sheffield
Sheffield
UK

Ali Gooya 🄳
University of Sheffield
Sheffield
UK

Jerry L. Prince 🄳
The Johns Hopkins University
Baltimore, MD
USA

ISSN 0302-9743   ISSN 1611-3349 (electronic)
Lecture Notes in Computer Science
ISBN 978-3-319-68126-9   ISBN 978-3-319-68127-6 (eBook)
DOI 10.1007/978-3-319-68127-6

Library of Congress Control Number: 2017955231

LNCS Sublibrary: SL6 – Image Processing, Computer Vision, Pattern Recognition, and Graphics

© Springer International Publishing AG 2017
This work is subject to copyright. All rights are reserved by the Publisher, whether the whole or part of the material is concerned, specifically the rights of translation, reprinting, reuse of illustrations, recitation, broadcasting, reproduction on microfilms or in any other physical way, and transmission or information storage and retrieval, electronic adaptation, computer software, or by similar or dissimilar methodology now known or hereafter developed.
The use of general descriptive names, registered names, trademarks, service marks, etc. in this publication does not imply, even in the absence of a specific statement, that such names are exempt from the relevant protective laws and regulations and therefore free for general use.
The publisher, the authors and the editors are safe to assume that the advice and information in this book are believed to be true and accurate at the date of publication. Neither the publisher nor the authors or the editors give a warranty, express or implied, with respect to the material contained herein or for any errors or omissions that may have been made. The publisher remains neutral with regard to jurisdictional claims in published maps and institutional affiliations.

Printed on acid-free paper

This Springer imprint is published by Springer Nature
The registered company is Springer International Publishing AG
The registered company address is: Gewerbestrasse 11, 6330 Cham, Switzerland

Preface

The MICCAI community needs data with known ground truth to develop, evaluate, and validate image analysis and reconstruction algorithms. Since synthetic data are ideally suited for this purpose, over the years, a full range of models underpinning image simulation and synthesis have been developed: (a) simplified mathematical models to test segmentation and registration algorithms; (b) detailed mechanistic models (top–down), which incorporate priors on the geometry and physics of image acquisition and formation processes; and (c) complex spatio temporal computational models of anatomical variability, organ physiology, or disease progression. Recently, cross-fertilization between image computing and machine learning gave rise to data-driven, phenomenological models (bottom–up) that stem from learning directly data associations across modalities, resolutions, etc. With this, not only has the application scope been expanded but the underlying model assumptions have also been refined to increasing levels of realism.

The goal of the Simulation and Synthesis in Medical Imaging (SASHIMI) Workshop is to gather all those interested in these problems in the same room, for the purpose of invigorating research and stimulating new ideas on how to best proceed and bring these two worlds together. The objectives were to: (a) hear from invited speakers in the areas of transfer learning and mechanistic models and cross-fertilize across fields; (b) bring together experts of synthesis (via phenomenological machine learning) and simulation (via explicit mechanistic models) to raise the state of the art; and (c) identify challenges and opportunities for further research. We also wanted to identify how we can best evaluate synthetic data and if we could collect benchmark data that can help the development of future algorithms.

Following the success from last year, the second SASHIMI[1] workshop was held in conjunction with the 20th International Conference on Medical Image Computing and Computer-Assisted Intervention (MICCAI 2017) as a satellite event in Quebec City, Quebec, Canada, on September 10, 2017. Submissions were solicited via a call for papers that was circulated by the MICCAI organizers, through known mailing lists (e.g., ImageWorld, MIUA) but also by directly e-mailing several colleagues and experts in the area. Each submission underwent a double-blind review by at least two members of the Program Committee consisting of researchers who actively contribute in the area. At the conclusion of the review process, 11 papers were accepted. Overall, the contributions span the following broad categories in alignment with the initial call for papers: cross modality (PET/MR, PET/CT, CT/MR, etc.) image synthesis, simulation and synthesis from large-scale image databases, automated techniques for quality assessment images, and several applications of image synthesis and simulation in medical imaging such as image interpolation and segmentation, image reconstruction, cell imaging, and blood flow. The accepted papers were divided into two general topics

---

[1] http://www.cistib.org/sashimi/.

of "Synthesis and Its Applications in Computational Medical Imaging" and "Simulation and Processing Approaches for Medical Imaging" and presented during two oral and one poster sessions, overall covering eight and three papers, respectively.

Finally, we would like to thank everyone who contributed to this second workshop: Helena Margarida Faria and Filipa Castro, members of the Organizing Committee, for their assistance; the authors for their contributions; the members of the Program Committee for their review work, promotion of the workshop, and general support; the invited speaker (Dr. Hugo Larochelle, Google Brain) for sharing his expertise and knowledge; and the MICCAI society for the general support.

August 2017

Sotirios A. Tsaftaris
Ali Gooya
Alejandro F. Frangi
Jerry L. Prince

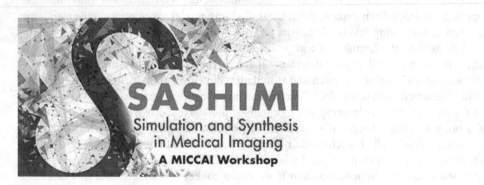

Organization

Workshop Chairs

Sotirios A. Tsaftaris	University of Edinburgh, UK
Ali Gooya	University of Sheffield, UK
Alejandro F. Frangi	University of Sheffield, UK
Jerry L. Prince	Johns Hopkins University, USA

Organizing Committee

Filipa Castro	University of Sheffield, UK
Helena Faria	University of Sheffield, UK

Program Committee

Martino Alessandrini	University of Bologna, Italy
Agis Chartsias	University of Edinburgh, UK
Sotirios A. Tsaftaris	University of Edinburgh, UK
M. Jorge Cardoso	University College London, UK
Tim Cootes	University of Manchester, UK
Marleen de Brujine	Erasmus University Medical Center, The Netherlands
Herve Delingette	Inria Sophia Antipolis, France
Dimitrios Fotiadis	University of Ioannina, Greece
Ali Gooya	University of Sheffield, UK
Daniel Herzka	John Hopkins University, USA
Ender Konukoglu	ETH Zurich, Switzerland
Hien V. Nguyen	Siemens Corporate Research, USA
Dzung L. Pham	National Institutes of Health, USA
Adityo Prakosa	John Hopkins University, USA
Snehashis Roy	National Institutes of Health, USA
Dinggang Shen	University of North Carolina, USA
François Varray	CREATIS, France
Devrim Unay	Izmir University of Economics, Turkey
Alistair Young	University of Auckland, New Zealand
Thomas Joyce	University of Edinburgh, UK
Yawen Huang	University of Sheffield, UK
Jonathan Mason	University of Edinburgh, UK

Contents

Synthesis and Its Applications in Computational Medical Imaging

Adversarial Image Synthesis for Unpaired Multi-modal Cardiac Data

Agisilaos Chartsias[1](✉), Thomas Joyce[1], Rohan Dharmakumar[2],
and Sotirios A. Tsaftaris[1]

[1] School of Engineering, Institute for Digital Communications,
University of Edinburgh, West Mains Road, Edinburgh EH9 3FB, UK
agis.chartsias@ed.ac.uk
[2] Cedars Sinai Medical Center, Los Angeles, CA, USA

Abstract. This paper demonstrates the potential for synthesis of medical images in one modality (e.g. MR) from images in another (e.g. CT) using a CycleGAN [24] architecture. The synthesis can be learned from unpaired images, and applied directly to expand the quantity of available training data for a given task. We demonstrate the application of this approach in synthesising cardiac MR images from CT images, using a dataset of MR and CT images coming from different patients. Since there can be no direct evaluation of the synthetic images, as no ground truth images exist, we demonstrate their utility by leveraging our synthetic data to achieve improved results in segmentation. Specifically, we show that training on both real and synthetic data increases accuracy by 15% compared to real data. Additionally, our synthetic data is of sufficient quality to be used alone to train a segmentation neural network, that achieves 95% of the accuracy of the same model trained on real data.

Keywords: Synthesis · MR · CT · Cardiac · Deep learning · GAN

1 Introduction

Medical imaging research has benefited significantly from the application of modern deep learning techniques. Yet, often the very best deep learning results outwith medical imaging are achieved when large labelled datasets are available. This is difficult in the medical setting, as medical data is often very sparsely labelled (generally requiring labelling by experts), expensive to obtain, and has to respect patient anonymity constraints. All of these factors make large labelled datasets rare in medical image analysis, and thus investigation into methods for mitigating this restriction are valuable.

When attempting to develop a model for a new task, it is common for only a limited quantity of labelled data in the modality of interest to exist. However, the same anatomy may have been imaged in other individuals and in other modalities, and then carefully labelled by experts. The fact that this labelled

---

A. Chartsias and T. Joyce—Contributed equally.

© Springer International Publishing AG 2017
S.A. Tsaftaris et al. (Eds.): SASHIMI 2017, LNCS 10557, pp. 3–13, 2017.
DOI: 10.1007/978-3-319-68127-6_1

data is not in the 'correct' modality means it is not immediately useful, but the ability to make use of these auxiliary labelled datasets would be extremely valuable, potentially enlarging the pool of labelled data many-fold.

In this paper we propose a pipeline for directly transforming auxiliary labelled data into the modality of interest (the "target modality"). We demonstrate that a small set of labelled data in the target modality can be used as a bootstrap, allowing us to convert labelled data from other modalities into the desired modality and expand the dataset. Additionally, this synthetic data consists of new examples not derived from existing examples, and potentially containing beneficial new anatomical and topological information from the auxiliary data. We show that this larger and more diverse dataset can then be used to train an improved model for the task at hand. Here, we demonstrate this for myocardial segmentation. However, as the data only needs to be of the same anatomy (not necessarily from the same individuals for example), the method can potentially expand the available training data for many tasks. Moreover, the method is especially suitable for cardiac use, as it does not require co-registered data.

The pipeline for our approach is as follows: firstly, we perform a view alignment step, transforming the auxiliary data so that the scale, position and viewing angle is broadly the same as in the target modality (Sect. 3.1). Secondly, we make use of a CycleGAN [24] architecture for unpaired image synthesis. This uses adversarial training to overcome the need for aligned pairs of images in the source and target modalities, and learns to transform data from one modality to the other. Once trained, we use the learned transformation to convert all the auxiliary data into synthetic data in the target modality (Sect. 3.2). A schematic overview of our approach is given in Fig. 1.

To evaluate this approach we apply our method to cardiac synthesis, generating cardiac MR images from cardiac CT images (Sect. 4). Directly quantitatively assessing the quality of synthetic data when no ground truth exists is very challenging. We demonstrate the synthetic data's utility by showing it significantly improves results in a segmentation task.

Specifically, this paper makes the following contributions: 1. Introduction of a flexible pipeline for transforming labelled data in auxiliary modalities into labelled data in the modality of interest. 2. A demonstration that augmenting real data with this synthetic data significantly improves performance in a segmentation task. 3. Comparison of our synthetic augmentation with standard augmentation, showing the synthesis approach to be favourable. 4. Demonstration of a recommended approach, which combines both synthesis and augmentation, and results in the best performance overall.

2   Previous Work

There has been very little previous work on learning-based methods for cardiac synthesis. Existing approaches have focused on combining electro-mechanical models of the heart's motion with template real images for generating image simulations [1, 14] and have been recently extended for simulation of pathologic

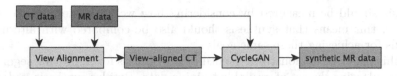

Fig. 1. A high-level schematic of the synthesis pipeline for the cardiac data. The Cycle-GAN also produces synthetic CT images but here we only use the synthetic MR.

from healthy cases [5] and for multimodal image simulation of both pathologic and healthy images in MR modalities [23].

Our work is based on learning a transformation function between images in order to transfer anatomical information from a source to a target modality. Similar methods have been proposed for cross-modal synthesis of brain images [4,7,10,17,21]. However, these are made possible by the availability of co-registered multimodal datasets, which allow a mapping from one modality to another to be directly learned using supervised techniques. In the cardiac domain, such registered multimodal datasets are harder to create. This is in part due to several unique challenges that cardiac data presents. Many of these difficulties result from the fact that the heart is an active moving muscle during the data acquisition session, and thus imaging it is more difficult than imaging the brain, or bones, which are essentially static relative to the body. In addition, the fact that the heart is moving makes it very difficult to produce co-registered images of the heart in different imaging modalities, and registration is often a complex non-linear post-processing step [18].

Cardiac synthesis methods have been explored for super-resolution (i.e. spatial up-sampling) in [12]. These methods can be learned by creating a low resolution version of a dataset, and then learning to synthesise the original resolution, again admitting a supervised approach. Recently, cardiac super-resolution has been enhanced by incorporating a shape prior in the learning process [13].

Furthermore, super-resolution has been coupled with cross-modal synthesis in a dictionary learning approach, with the addition of unpaired data in the learning process to improve the quality of results [8], proposing a weakly supervised learning approach. Unpaired data has also been used for cross-modal synthesis in an optimisation scheme [22], treating the problem as unsupervised learning. However, [22] focuses only on brain images, and does not address cardiac.

Unsupervised learning, for example learning image transformations with no ground-truth target images, has been revolutionalised by the introduction of adversarial training of neural networks [6,15]. Adversarial learning was used for image style transformation in [24], and this method is directly applicable to cardiac data, where there is a lack of paired data.

Although synthesis offers a flexible approach that can be directly applied to expand available data, it is still important to weigh synthesis up, critically, against other approaches. Synthetic data has been used previously to improve segmentation [9] and classification algorithms [20], and, as there is no direct way to measure accuracy when ground truth images do not exist, the value of synthesis should be measured by considering how well it achieves these aims. However, this means that synthesis should also be compared with alternative methods for achieving these same goals.

In this paper we demonstrate the utility of synthesis for improving segmentation via enlarging the set of available training data. Besides synthesis, a dataset can also be expanded using simple geometric augmentation, for example by rotating and reflecting the images. Although simple transformation based augmentation is commonly used to improve results on cardiac segmentation [19,23], this approach produces derivative examples, and does not benefit from the existence of auxiliary data, which could potentially provide additional real anatomical examples. In our experiments (Sect. 4) we directly compare this standard data augmentation with our synthesis approach, and, as the approaches are not mutually exclusive, also explore combining both approaches.

3   Method Details

We now give step-by-step details of our method, describing the view alignment, the training of the CycleGAN and the generation of the synthetic data.

3.1   View Alignment

In the view alignment step we make the CT and MR image sets broadly similar in terms of structure. Specifically, we aim to make the layout of the images (the position and size of the anatomy for example) not informative as to the dataset from which the image came. Preventing this is important in order to ensure the adversarial training is effective, otherwise the discriminator may learn to differentiate between real and synthetic data by attending to structural differences, rather than intensity statistics. However, the alignment only needs to be approximate, and any simple registration approach should suffice. Here we make use of the multiple labels on the data, using them to approximate the affine transformation that, for a given MR and CT volume, when applied to the CT volume, maximises alignment with the MR volume. After this crude alignment, any points in the new CT volume that correspond to points outside of the original CT volume are set to 0. Additionally, any points in the MR volume that correspond to points outside of the original CT volume are also set to 0. This again is performed to make the volumes structurally similar, to aid the adversarial training.

3.2   Transform Learning with CycleGAN

Since the images are not paired, learning to transform from MR to CT is not straightforward. However, a recent adversarial approach to this difficult task is the CycleGAN [24]: an adversarialy trained deep network which simultaneously learns transformations between two datasets containing the same information,

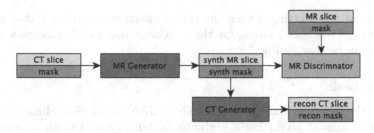

Fig. 2. Unfolded CycleGAN [24] training for CT to MR synthesis: a CT image with its segmentation mask is mapped to a synthetic MR and mask by a generator network $F : [CT, Mask] \rightarrow [MR, Mask]$. An MR discriminator then tries to discriminate real from synthetic MR. The CT and Mask are also reconstructed form the synthetic MR by a second generator network $G : [MR, Mask] \rightarrow [CT, Mask]$, which aims to reconstruct the original CT exactly. The generator learns both by trying to fool the discriminator, and by minimising the discrepancy between the real CT and its reconstruction.

but differently represented. It is powerful since it does not require paired training data, but instead learns via the use of both a discriminator and a cycle loss.

Specifically, a transform $F : A \rightarrow B$ is learned from dataset A to dataset B to produce synthetic B data y^B from real A data x^A, i.e. $y^B = F(x^A)$. Transform F aims to fool a discriminator D_B, which is simultaneously learning to discriminate between real and synthetic B data. Additionally, the synthetic B data is then transformed back into its original modality by a second learned transform $G :$ $B \rightarrow A$ going in the other direction $x^A = G(y^B)$. This allows for an additional cost to be included in the training: data mapped from A to B, then back to A, should be as close as possible to the original A. That is $G(F(x^A))$ should be equal to x^A. This cycle loss gives the model its name.

In our case, the CycleGAN learns to transform a CT image into a synthetic MR image that cannot be recognised as synthetic by a discriminator network. At the same time, the synthetic MR image must be able to be accurately converted back into a CT image, as similar as possible to the original CT image, via another learned transformation. Thus, the synthetic MR image, whilst appearing realistic, must also retain relevant information from the CT. This encourages the synthetic MR to contain the same anatomy as is present in the input CT.

Adversarial training of deep neural networks is a challenging task, sensitive to many variables, and increasing the accessibility of the approach is an active area of research [2,3]. Initially, we applied the CycleGAN directly to the MR and CT images. However, we found that although the resulting images were promising in terms of realism, the myocardium in the synthetic image was often not in the same place as in the input image. As a result, our synthetic MR data had no accurate labels, as we could not assume the label was the same as in the input image. To mitigate this issue we included both the mask of the myocardium and the image as two channel inputs to the CycleGAN, such that it learned to transform CT images and their corresponding myocardium segmentation mask into realistic MR images and corresponding segmentation masks. This did not stop the anatomy shifting during the transformation, but meant that we still had accurate (synthetic) labels for the synthetic images. A schematic of this approach can be seen in Fig. 2.

3.3 Synthesis

We apply the mapping learned with the CycleGAN to the view-aligned CT data and the CT masks, producing a synthetic MR image and mask for every CT image in the dataset. The result is a synthetic labelled data set of MR cardiac images, which can be used for any task of interest.

4 Experiments

In this section we examine the effect of synthetic results in the accuracy of myocardium segmentation. We train a segmentation model, detailed in Sect. 4.1, on various combinations of synthetic and real data, with and without augmentation and report the dice coefficient on 3-fold cross validation.

4.1 Segmentation

To segment the images, we train a neural network with an architecture similar to the U-Net [16]. Specifically, the network consists of 3 downsample and 3 upsample blocks with skip connections between each block of equal size filters. This architecture was chosen as similar fully convolutional networks have been shown to achieve state of the art results in various segmentation tasks, including cardiac, and U-Net is a standard benchmark approach. Here we have not specifically optimised the architecture or hyperparameters for the segmentation task being considered, since the aim is to evaluate the synthetic results. Our model is implemented in Keras[1] and trained using Adam [11] with batch-size 16 and an early stopping criterion, based on the validation data, to avoid overfitting.

4.2 Data

We use 40 anonymised volumes, of which 20 are cardiac CT/CTA and 20 are cardiac MRI, kindly made available by the authors of [25,26]. The CT/CTA data were acquired at Shanghai Shuguang Hospital, China, using routine cardiac CT angiography. The slices were acquired in the axial view. The inplane resolution is about 0.78×0.78 mm and the average slice thickness is 1.60 mm. The MRI data were acquired at St. Thomas hospital and Royal Brompton Hospital, London, UK, using 3D balanced steady state free precession (b-SSFP) sequences, with about 2 mm acquisition resolution at each direction and reconstructed (resampled) into about 1 mm. The data contains static 3D images, acquired at different time points relative to the systole and diastole. All the data has manual segmentation of the seven whole heart substructures. However, in our segmentation experiments we only use the labels for the myocardium of the left ventricle.

---

[1] https://keras.io.

4.3 Data Preprocessing

We centered the anatomy (the bounding box of the labeled anatomical regions) within the MR volumes, and trimmed each volume to 232×232, padding with 0s where necessary, but maintaining the native resolution. Then, for each volume, we clipped the top 1% of pixel values and re-scaled the values to $[-1, 1]$. Finally, we removed slices that did not contain myocardium, resulting in 20 volumes with an average of 41 slices per volume (816 slices in total). For the cardiac CT data no centering or trimming was necessary, as the data is aligned with the MR data in the view alignment step of Sect. 3.1. However, we again clipped the top 1% of values, and scaled the values to $[-1, 1]$.

4.4 Experiment Details

Below we detail the five experiments we used to evaluate the quality of the synthesised cardiac MR data. We repeated all experiments on three different splits of the data, each time training a CycleGAN on 15 MR and 15 CT volumes, and then training the segmentation network described in Sect. 4.1. In every split, the 5 MR volumes used for testing the segmentation network were excluded, as were the 5 CT volumes which were aligned with them in the view alignment step. Thus the final test volumes have not been used anywhere in the pipeline. Out of the remaining 15 MR volumes, we used 10 for training and 5 for validation.

Real: Firstly, as a baseline we train the segmentation network on 10 real MR volumes, using the other 5 MR volumes for validation, and obtain a mean dice coefficient of 0.613 on the test set.

Synthetic: Secondly, to directly evaluate the quality of the synthetic data, we train the segmentation network on 10 synthetic volumes, validating on 5 synthetic volumes. We then test the final model on the 5 real MR volumes and obtained a dice coefficient of 0.580.

Real and Synthetic: Next we combine the real and synthetic data and train our segmentation network on a total of 25 volumes (10 real and 15 synthetic), again using 5 real volumes for validation. This combined training gives a performance gain of ~15% compared to training on real data alone.

Augmented Real: Next we augment the real data using horizontal and vertical flips generating a total training set of 25 volumes (10 real 15 flipped) to allow direct comparison with synthetic augmentation.

Augmented Real and Synthetic: Finally, we combine the real and synthetic training data, and also use horizontal and vertical flips to expand the data to double the size. This results in 50 training volumes, and we again use 5 real volumes for validation during training.

4.5 Results

All results are presented side-by-side in Table 1. In addition, in Fig. 3 we provide examples of our synthetic results. The first observation is that using just the synthetic data is almost as good as using the real data, in terms of resulting

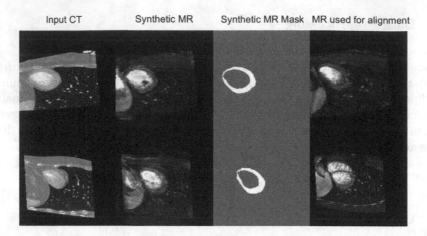

Fig. 3. Two examples of MR synthesis. From left to right it is shown, the real CT image, the resulting synthetic MR image, the synthetic segmentation mask and finally the real MR image of the volume to which the real CT volume was aligned in the view alignment step. Note that the shape and position of the myocardium is similar but not identical between the CT input and corresponding synthetic MR output. Also, observe that in the upper row the synthetic data contains a dark artifact within the ventricle.

Table 1. Dice scores for U-Nets trained on various data combinations. In all cases the model is evaluated on real MR images.

Training data	Split 1	Split 2	Split 3	Average	Relative to real
Just synthetic	0.553	0.516	0.672	0.580	0.946
Just real	0.584	0.613	0.642	0.613	1.000
Augmented real	0.632	0.685	0.711	0.676	1.103
Real and synthetic	**0.657**	0.699	**0.757**	0.704	1.148
Augmented real and synthetic	0.650	**0.738**	0.748	**0.712**	**1.161**

segmentation, only resulting in a 5% loss of accuracy and this difference is not statistically significant at the 5% level. This is likely the result of small errors present in the synthetic images. Next, it is informative to compare real data with standard augmentations against the combined real and synthetic data. In both cases the segmentation algorithm was trained on 25 volumes, including the same 10 real volumes, and both approaches improve the final segmentation accuracy with synthetic and geometric augmentation leading to 14.8% and 10.3% improvements respectively. Finally, when the real and synthetic data is combined, and geometric augmentations are also applied, the greatest improvement is seen, with a 16.1% increase in accuracy over the baseline.

The difference in performance between the real and synthetic data, and just the real data is significant at the 5% level, as is the difference between the real and synthetic data and the augmented real data. Further, adding augmentation to the real and synthetic data does not lead to a statistically significant improvement.

5   Discussion and Conclusion

We have demonstrated that it is possible to produce synthetic cardiac data from unpaired images coming from different individuals. Moreover, we demonstrate that these synthetic images are accurate enough to be of significant benefit for further tasks, either used alone or to enlarge existing data sets. Specifically, we have shown that it is possible to produce synthetic cardiac MR images from cardiac CT images, and that these images can be used to improve the accuracy of a segmentation algorithm by 16% when used in combination with standard geometric augmentation techniques. We also demonstrated that the synthetic data alone was sufficient to train a segmentation algorithm only 5% less accurate than the same algorithm trained entirely on real data.

As can be seen in the results, the largest gains are made when the synthetic data is included in the training set, suggesting that new anatomy, containing additional examples of real structure and natural local variations, being introduced from the auxiliary data is most beneficial for improving results.

Acknowledgements. This work was supported in part by the US National Institutes of Health (2R01HL091989-05) and UK EPSRC (EP/P022928/1). We thank NVIDIA for donating a Titan X GPU.

References

1. Alessandrini, M., De Craene, M., Bernard, O., Giffard-Roisin, S., Allain, P., Waechter-Stehle, I., Weese, J., Saloux, E., Delingette, H., Sermesant, M.: A pipeline for the generation of realistic 3D synthetic echocardiographic sequences: methodology and open-access database. IEEE TMI **34**(7), 1436–1451 (2015)
2. Arjovsky, M., Chintala, S., Bottou, L.: Wasserstein gan. preprint arXiv:1701.07875 (2017)
3. Berthelot, D., Schumm, T., Metz, L.: BEGAN: Boundary Equilibrium Generative Adversarial Networks. preprint arXiv:1703.10717 (2017)
4. Cordier, N., Delingette, H., Lê, M., Ayache, N.: Extended modality propagation: image synthesis of pathological cases. IEEE TMI **35**(12), 2598–2608 (2016)
5. Duchateau, N., Sermesant, M., Delingette, H., Ayache, N.: Model-based generation of large databases of cardiac images: synthesis of pathological cine MR sequences from real healthy cases. IEEE TMI (99) (2017). doi:10.1109/TMI.2017.2714343
6. Goodfellow, I., et al.: Generative adversarial nets. In: NIPS, pp. 2672–2680 (2014)
7. Huang, Y., Beltrachini, L., Shao, L., Frangi, A.F.: Geometry regularized joint dictionary learning for cross-modality image synthesis in magnetic resonance imaging. In: Tsaftaris, S.A., Gooya, A., Frangi, A.F., Prince, J.L. (eds.) SASHIMI 2016. LNCS, vol. 9968, pp. 118–126. Springer, Cham (2016). doi:10.1007/978-3-319-46630-9_12

8. Huang, Y., Shao, L., Frangi, A.F.: Simultaneous super-resolution and cross-modality synthesis of 3D medical images using weakly-supervised joint convolutional sparse coding. preprint arXiv:1705.02596 (2017)

9. Iglesias, J.E., Konukoglu, E., Zikic, D., Glocker, B., Van Leemput, K., Fischl, B.: Is synthesizing MRI contrast useful for inter-modality analysis? In: Mori, K., Sakuma, I., Sato, Y., Barillot, C., Navab, N. (eds.) MICCAI 2013. LNCS, vol. 8149, pp. 631–638. Springer, Heidelberg (2013). doi:10.1007/978-3-642-40811-3_79

10. Jog, A., Carass, A., Roy, S., Pham, D.L., Prince, J.L.: Random forest regression for magnetic resonance image synthesis. Med. Image Anal. **35**, 475–488 (2017)

11. Kingma, D., Ba, J.: Adam: a method for stochastic optimization. preprint arXiv:1412.6980 (2014)

12. Oktay, O., et al.: Multi-input cardiac image super-resolution using convolutional neural networks. In: Ourselin, S., Joskowicz, L., Sabuncu, M.R., Unal, G., Wells, W. (eds.) MICCAI 2016. LNCS, vol. 9902, pp. 246–254. Springer, Cham (2016). doi:10.1007/978-3-319-46726-9_29

13. Oktay, O., Ferrante, E., Kamnitsas, K., Heinrich, M., Bai, W., Caballero, J., Guerrero, R., Cook, S., de Marvao, A., O'Regan, D.: Anatomically constrained neural networks (ACNN): application to cardiac image enhancement and segmentation. preprint arXiv:1705.08302 (2017)

14. Prakosa, A., Sermesant, M., Delingette, H., Marchesseau, S., Saloux, E., Allain, P., Villain, N., Ayache, N.: Generation of synthetic but visually realistic time series of cardiac images combining a biophysical model and clinical images. IEEE TMI **32**(1), 99–109 (2013)

15. Radford, A., Metz, L., Chintala, S.: Unsupervised representation learning with deep convolutional generative adversarial networks. preprint arXiv:1511.06434 (2015)

16. Ronneberger, O., Fischer, P., Brox, T.: U-Net: convolutional networks for biomedical image segmentation. In: Navab, N., Hornegger, J., Wells, W.M., Frangi, A.F. (eds.) MICCAI 2015. LNCS, vol. 9351, pp. 234–241. Springer, Cham (2015). doi:10.1007/978-3-319-24574-4_28

17. Sevetlidis, V., Giuffrida, M.V., Tsaftaris, S.A.: Whole image synthesis using a deep encoder-decoder network. In: Tsaftaris, S.A., Gooya, A., Frangi, A.F., Prince, J.L. (eds.) SASHIMI 2016. LNCS, vol. 9968, pp. 127–137. Springer, Cham (2016). doi:10.1007/978-3-319-46630-9_13

18. Tavakoli, V., Amini, A.A.: A survey of shaped-based registration and segmentation techniques for cardiac images. Comput. Vis. Image Underst. **117**(9), 966–989 (2013)

19. Tran, P.V.: A fully convolutional neural network for cardiac segmentation in short-axis MRI. preprint arXiv:1604.00494 (2016)

20. van Tulder, G., de Bruijne, M.: Why does synthesized data improve multi-sequence classification? In: Navab, N., Hornegger, J., Wells, W.M., Frangi, A.F. (eds.) MICCAI 2015. LNCS, vol. 9349, pp. 531–538. Springer, Cham (2015). doi:10.1007/978-3-319-24553-9_65

21. Van Nguyen, H., Zhou, K., Vemulapalli, R.: Cross-domain synthesis of medical images using efficient location-sensitive deep network. In: Navab, N., Hornegger, J., Wells, W.M., Frangi, A.F. (eds.) MICCAI 2015. LNCS, vol. 9349, pp. 677–684. Springer, Cham (2015). doi:10.1007/978-3-319-24553-9_83

22. Vemulapalli, R., Van Nguyen, H., Kevin Zhou, S.: Unsupervised cross-modal synthesis of subject-specific scans. In: IEEE ICCV, pp. 630–638 (2015)

23. Zhou, Y., Giffard-Roisin, S., De Craene, M., D'hooge, J., Alessandrini, M., Friboulet, D., Sermesant, M., Bernard, O.: A framework for the generation of realistic synthetic cardiac ultrasound and magnetic resonance imaging sequences from the same virtual patients. IEEE TMI (99) (2017). doi:10.1109/TMI.2017.2708159
24. Zhu, J.: Unpaired image-to-image translation using cycle-consistent adversarial networks. preprint arXiv:1703.10593 (2017)
25. Zhuang, X., Rhode, K.S., Razavi, R.S., Hawkes, D.J., Ourselin, S.: A registration-based propagation framework for automatic whole heart segmentation of cardiac MRI. IEEE TMI **29**(9), 1612–1625 (2010)
26. Zhuang, X., Shen, J.: Multi-scale patch and multi-modality atlases for whole heart segmentation of MRI. Med. Image Anal. **31**, 77–87 (2016)

Deep MR to CT Synthesis Using Unpaired Data

Jelmer M. Wolterink[1](✉), Anna M. Dinkla[2], Mark H.F. Savenije[2],
Peter R. Seevinck[1], Cornelis A.T. van den Berg[2], and Ivana Išgum[1]

[1] Image Sciences Institute, University Medical Center Utrecht,
Utrecht, The Netherlands
`j.m.wolterink@umcutrecht.nl`
[2] Department of Radiotherapy, University Medical Center Utrecht,
Utrecht, The Netherlands

Abstract. MR-only radiotherapy treatment planning requires accurate
MR-to-CT synthesis. Current deep learning methods for MR-to-CT synthesis depend on pairwise aligned MR and CT training images of the
same patient. However, misalignment between paired images could lead
to errors in synthesized CT images. To overcome this, we propose to
train a generative adversarial network (GAN) with unpaired MR and CT
images. A GAN consisting of two synthesis convolutional neural networks
(CNNs) and two discriminator CNNs was trained with cycle consistency
to transform 2D brain MR image slices into 2D brain CT image slices
and vice versa. Brain MR and CT images of 24 patients were analyzed.
A quantitative evaluation showed that the model was able to synthesize
CT images that closely approximate reference CT images, and was able
to outperform a GAN model trained with paired MR and CT images.

Keywords: Deep learning · Radiotherapy · Treatment planning · CT
synthesis · Generative adversarial networks

1 Introduction

Radiotherapy treatment planning requires a magnetic resonance (MR) volume
for segmentation of tumor volume and organs at risk, as well as a spatially corresponding computed tomography (CT) volume for dose planning. Separate acquisition of these volumes is time-consuming, costly and a burden to the patient.
Furthermore, voxel-wise spatial alignment between MR and CT images may be
compromised, requiring accurate registration of MR and CT volumes. Hence, to
circumvent separate CT acquisition, a range of methods have been proposed for
MR-only radiotherapy treatment planning in which a substitute or synthetic CT
image is derived from the available MR image [2].

Previously proposed methods have used convolutional neural networks
(CNNs) for CT synthesis in the brain [4] and pelvic area [8]. These CNNs are
trained by minimization of voxel-wise differences with respect to reference CT
volumes that are rigidly aligned with the input MR images. However, slight
voxel-wise misalignment of MR and CT images may lead to synthesis of blurred

© Springer International Publishing AG 2017
S.A. Tsaftaris et al. (Eds.): SASHIMI 2017, LNCS 10557, pp. 14–23, 2017.
DOI: 10.1007/978-3-319-68127-6_2

Paired data   Unpaired data

MR

CT

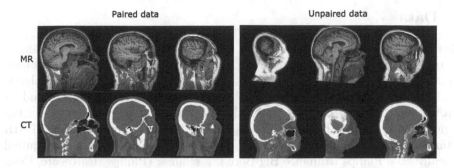

Fig. 1. *Left* When training with paired data, MR and CT slices that are simultaneously provided to the network correspond to the same patient at the same anatomical location. *Right* When training with unpaired data, MR and CT slices that are simultaneously provided to the network belong to different patients at different locations in the brain.

images. To address this, Nie et al. [9] proposed to combine the voxel-wise loss with an image-wise adversarial loss in a generative adversarial network (GAN) [3]. In this GAN, the synthesis CNN competes with a discriminator CNN that aims to distinguish synthetic images from real CT images. The discriminator CNN provides feedback to the synthesis CNN based on the overall quality of the synthesized CT images.

Although the GAN method by Nie et al. [9] addresses the issue of image misalignment by incorporating an image-wise loss, it still contains a voxel-wise loss component requiring a training set of paired MR and CT volumes. In practice, such a training set may be hard to obtain. Furthermore, given the scarcity of training data, it may be beneficial to utilize additional MR or CT training volumes from patients who were scanned for different purposes and who have not necessarily been imaged using both modalities. The use of unpaired MR and CT training data would relax many of the requirements of current deep learning-based CT synthesis systems (Fig. 1).

Recently, methods have been proposed to train image-to-image translation CNNs with unpaired natural images, namely DualGAN [11] and CycleGAN [12]. Like the methods proposed in [4,8,9], these CNNs translate an image from one domain to another domain. Unlike these methods, the loss function during training depends solely on the overall quality of the synthesized image as determined by an adversarial discriminator network. To prevent the synthesis CNN from generating images that look real but bear little similarity to the input image, cycle consistency is enforced. That is, an additional CNN is trained to translate the synthesized image back to the original domain and the difference between this reconstructed image and the original image is added as a regularization term during training.

Here, we use a CycleGAN model to synthesize brain CT images from brain MR images. We show that training with pairs of spatially aligned MR and CT images of the same patients is not necessary for deep learning-based CT synthesis.

2   Data

This study included brain MR and CT images of 24 patients that were scanned for radiotherapy treatment planning of brain tumors. MR and CT images were acquired on the same day in radiation treatment position using a thermoplastic mask for immobilization. Patients with heavy dental artefacts on CT and/or MR were excluded. T1 3D MR (repetition time 6.98 ms, echo time 3.14 ms, flip angle 8°) images were obtained with dual flex coils on a Philips Ingenia 1.5T MR scanner (Philips Healthcare, Best, The Netherlands). CT images were acquired helically on a Philips Brilliance Big Bore CT scanner (Philips Healthcare, Best, The Netherlands) with 120 kVp and 450 mAs. To allow voxel-wise comparison of synthetic and reference CT images, MR and CT images of the same patient were aligned using rigid registration based on mutual information following a clinical procedure. This registration did not correct for local misalignment (Fig. 2). CT images had a resolution of $1.00 \times 0.90 \times 0.90$ mm^3 and were resampled to the same voxel size as the MR, namely $1.00 \times 0.87 \times 0.87$ mm^3. Each volume had $183 \times 288 \times 288$ voxels. A head region mask excluding surrounding air was obtained in the CT image and propagated to the MR image.

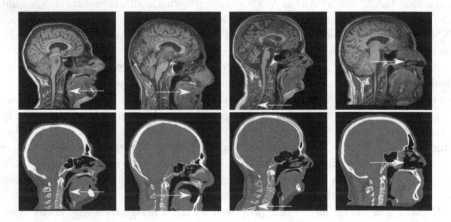

Fig. 2. Examples showing local misalignment between MR and CT images after rigid registration using mutual information. Although the skull is generally well-aligned, misalignments may occur in the throat, mouth, vertebrae, and nasal cavities.

3   Methods

The CycleGAN model proposed by Zhu et al. and used in this work contains a forward and a backward cycle (Fig. 3) [12].

The forward cycle consists of three separate CNNs. First, network Syn_{CT} is trained to translate an input MR image I_{MR} into a CT image. Second, network Syn_{MR} is trained to translate a synthesized CT image $Syn_{CT}(I_{MR})$ back into an MR image. Third, network Dis_{CT} is trained to discriminate between synthesized

$Syn_{CT}(I_{MR})$ and real CT images I_{CT}. Each of these three neural networks has a different goal. While Dis_{CT} aims to distinguish synthesized CT images from real CT images, network Syn_{CT} tries to prevent this by synthesizing images that cannot be distinguished from real CT images. These images should be translated back to the MR domain by network Syn_{MR} so that the original image is reconstructed from $Syn_{CT}(I_{MR})$ as accurately as possible.

To improve training stability, the backward cycle is also trained, translating CT images into MR images and back into CT images. For synthesis, this model uses the same CNNs Syn_{CT} and Syn_{MR}. In addition, it contains a discriminator network Dis_{MR} that aims to distinguish synthesized MR images from real MR images.

The adversarial goals of the synthesis and discriminator networks are reflected in their loss functions. The discriminator Dis_{CT} aims to predict the label 1 for real CT images and the label 0 for synthesized CT images. Hence, the discriminator Dis_{CT} tries to minimize

$$\mathcal{L}_{CT} = (1 - Dis_{CT}(I_{CT}))^2 + Dis_{CT}(Syn_{CT}(I_{MR}))^2 \qquad (1)$$

for MR images I_{MR} and CT images I_{CT}. At the same time, synthesis network Syn_{CT} tries to maximize this loss by synthesizing images that cannot be distinguished from real CT images.

Similarly, the discriminator Dis_{MR} aims to predict the label 1 for real MR images and the label 0 for synthesized MR images. Hence, the loss function for MR synthesis that Dis_{MR} aims to minimize and Syn_{MR} aims to maximize is defined as

$$\mathcal{L}_{MR} = (1 - Dis_{MR}(I_{MR}))^2 + Dis_{MR}(Syn_{MR}(I_{CT}))^2 \qquad (2)$$

To enforce bidirectional cycle consistency during training, additional loss terms are defined as the difference between original and reconstructed images,

$$\mathcal{L}_{Cycle} = ||Syn_{MR}(Syn_{CT}(I_{MR})) - I_{MR}||_1 + ||Syn_{CT}(Syn_{MR}(I_{CT})) - I_{CT}||_1. \qquad (3)$$

During training, this term is weighted by a parameter λ and added to the loss functions for Syn_{CT} and Syn_{MR}.

3.1   CNN Architectures

The PyTorch implementation provided by the authors of [12] was used in all experiments[1]. This implementation performs voxel regression and image classification in 2D images. Here, experiments were performed using 2D sagittal image slices (Fig. 1). We provide a brief description of the synthesis and discriminator CNNs. Further implementation details are provided in [12].

The network architectures of Syn_{CT} and Syn_{MR} are identical. They are 2D fully convolutional networks with two strided convolution layers, nine residual

---

[1] https://github.com/junyanz/pytorch-CycleGAN-and-pix2pix.

Forward cycle

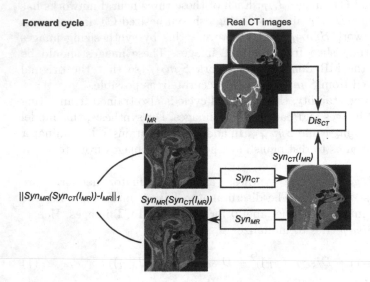

Backward cycle

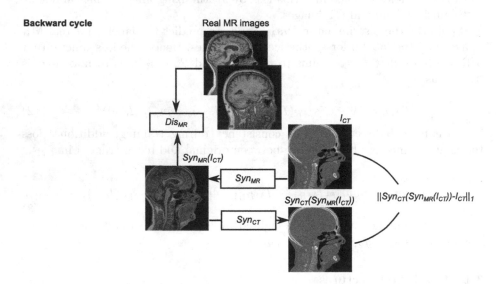

Fig. 3. The CycleGAN model consists of a forward cycle and a backward cycle. In the forward cycle, a synthesis network Syn_{CT} is trained to translate an input MR image I_{MR} into a CT image, network Syn_{MR} is trained to translate the resulting CT image back into an MR image that approximates the original MR image, and Dis_{CT} discriminates between real and synthesized CT images. In the backward cycle, Syn_{MR} synthesizes MR images from input CT images, Syn_{CT} reconstructs the input CT image from the synthesized image, and Dis_{MR} discriminates between real and synthesized MR images.

blocks and two fractionally strided convolution layers, based on the architecture proposed in [6] and used in [12]. Hence, the CNN takes input images of size 256×256 pixels and predicts output images of the same size.

Networks Dis_{CT} and Dis_{MR} also use the same architecture. This architecture does not provide one prediction for the full 256×256 pixel image, but instead uses a fully convolutional architecture to classify overlapping 70×70 image patches as real or fake [5]. This way, the CNN can better focus on high-frequency information that may distinguish real from synthesized images.

3.2 Evaluation

Real and synthesized CT images were compared using the mean absolute error

$$MAE = \frac{1}{N} \sum_{i=1}^{N} |I_{CT}(i) - Syn_{CT}(I_{MR}(i))|, \tag{4}$$

where i iterates over aligned voxels in the real and synthesized CT images. Note that this was based on the prior alignment of I_{MR} and I_{CT}. In addition, agreement was evaluated using the peak-signal-to-noise-ratio (PSNR) as proposed in [8,9] as

$$PSNR = 20 \log_{10} \frac{4095}{MSE}, \tag{5}$$

where MSE is the mean-squared error, i.e. $\frac{1}{N} \sum_{i=1}^{N} (I_{CT}(i) - Syn_{CT}(I_{MR}(i)))^2$. The MAE and PSNR were computed within a head region mask determined in both the CT and MR that excludes any surrounding air.

4 Experiments and Results

The 24 data sets were separated into a training set containing MR and CT volumes of 18 patients and a separate test set containing MR and corresponding reference CT volumes of 6 patients.

Each MR or CT volume contained 183 sagittal 2D image slices. These were resampled to 256×256 pixel images with 256 grayscale values uniformly distributed in $[-600, 1400]$ HU for CT and $[0, 3500]$ for MR. This put image values in the same range as in [12], so that the default value of $\lambda = 10$ was used to weigh cycle consistency loss. To augment the number of training samples, each image was padded to 286×286 pixels and sub-images of 256×256 pixels were randomly cropped during training. The model was trained using Adam [7] for 100 epochs with a fixed learning rate of 0.0002, and 100 epochs in which the learning rate was linearly reduced to zero. Model training took 52 h on a single NVIDIA Titan X GPU. MR to CT synthesis with a trained model took around 10 s.

Figure 4 shows an example MR input image, the synthesized CT image obtained by the model and the corresponding reference CT image. The model

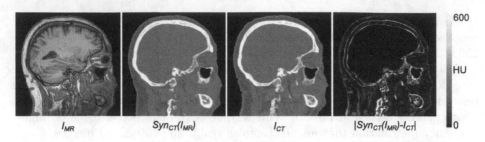

I_{MR} $Syn_{CT}(I_{MR})$ I_{CT} $|Syn_{CT}(I_{MR})-I_{CT}|$

Fig. 4. *From left to right* Input MR image, synthesized CT image, reference real CT image, and absolute error between real and synthesized CT image.

has learned to differentiate between different structures with similar intensity values in MR but not in CT, such as bone, ventricular fluid and air. The difference image shows the absolute error between the synthesized and real CT image. Differences are least pronounced in the soft brain tissue, and most in bone structures, such as the eye socket, the vertebrae and the jaw. This may be partly due to the reduced image quality in the neck area and misalignment between the MR image and the reference CT image. Table 1 shows a quantitative comparison between real CT and synthesized CT images in the test set. MAE and PSNR values show high consistency among the different test images.

To compare unpaired training with conventional paired training, an additional synthesis CNN with the same architecture as Syn_{CT} was trained using paired MR and CT image slices. For this, we used the implementation of [5] which, like [9], combines voxel-wise loss with adversarial feedback from a discriminator network. This discriminator network had the same architecture as Dis_{CT}. A paired t-test on the results in Table 1 showed that agreement with the reference CT images was significantly lower ($p < 0.05$) for images obtained using this model than for images obtained using the unpaired model. Figure 5

Table 1. Mean absolute error (MAE) values in HU and peak-signal-to-noise ratio (PSNR) between synthesized and real CT images when training with paired or unpaired data.

	MAE		PSNR	
	Unpaired	Paired	Unpaired	Paired
Patient 1	70.3	86.2	31.1	29.3
Patient 2	76.2	98.8	32.1	30.1
Patient 3	75.5	96.9	32.9	30.1
Patient 4	75.2	86.0	32.9	31.7
Patient 5	72.0	81.7	32.3	31.2
Patient 6	73.0	87.0	32.5	30.9
Average ± SD	73.7 ± 2.3	89.4 ± 6.8	32.3 ± 0.7	30.6 ± 0.9

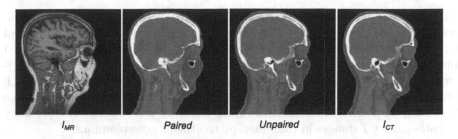

Fig. 5. *From left to right* Input MR image, synthesized CT image with paired training, synthesized CT image with unpaired training, reference real CT image.

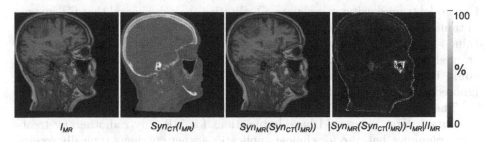

Fig. 6. *From left to right* Input MR image, synthesized CT image, reconstructed MR image, and relative error between the input and reconstructed MR image.

shows a visual comparison of results obtained with unpaired and paired training data. The image obtained with paired training data is more blurry and contains a high-intensity artifact in the neck.

During training, cycle consistency is explicitly imposed in both directions. Hence, an MR image that is translated to the CT domain should be successfully translated back to the MR domain. Figure 6 shows an MR image, a synthesized CT image and the reconstructed MR image. The difference map shows that although there are errors with respect to the original image, these are very small and homogeneously distributed. Relative differences are largest at the contour of the head and in air, where intensity values are low. The reconstructed MR image is remarkably similar to the original MR image.

5   Discussion and Conclusion

We have shown that a CNN can be trained to synthesize a CT image from an MR image using unpaired and unaligned MR and CT training images. In contrast to previous work, the model learns to synthesize realistically-looking images guided only by the performance of an adversarial discriminator network and the similarity of back-transformed output images to the original input image.

Quantitative evaluation using an independent test set of six images showed that the average correspondence between synthetic CT and reference CT images was 73.7 ± 2.3 HU (MAE) and 32.3 ± 0.7 (PSNR). In comparison, Nie et al. reported an MAE of 92.5 ± 13.9 HU and a PSNR of 27.6 ± 1.3 [9], and Han et al. reported an MAE of 84.8 ± 17.3 HU [4]. However, these studies used different data sets with different anatomical coverage, making a direct comparison infeasible. Furthermore, slight misalignments between reference MR and CT images, and thus between synthesized CT and reference CT, may have a large effect on quantitative evaluation. In future work, we will evaluate the accuracy of synthesized CT images in radiotherapy treatment dose planning.

Yi et al. showed that a model using cycle consistency for unpaired data can in some cases outperform a GAN-model on paired data [11]. Similarly, we found that in our test data sets, the model trained using unpaired data outperformed the model trained using paired data. Qualitative analysis showed that CT images obtained by the model trained with unpaired data looked more realistic, contained less artifacts and contained less blurring than those obtained by the model trained with paired data. This was reflected in the quantitative analysis. This could be due to misalignment between MR and CT images (Fig. 2), which is ignored when training with unpaired data.

The results indicate that image synthesis CNNs can be trained using unaligned data. This could have implications for MR-only radiotherapy treatment planning, but also for clinical applications where patients typically receive only one scan of a single anatomical region. In such scenarios, paired data is scarce, but there are many single acquisitions of different modalities. Possible applications are synthesis between MR images acquired at different field strengths [1], or between CT images acquired at different dose levels [10].

Although the CycleGAN implementation used in the current study was developed for natural images, synthesis was successfully performed in 2D medical images. In future work, we will investigate whether 3D information as present in MR and CT images can further improve performance. Nonetheless, the current results already showed that the synthesis network was able to efficiently translate structures with complex 3D appearance, such as vertebrae and bones.

The results in this study were obtained using a model that was trained with MR and CT images of the same patients. These images were rigidly registered to allow a voxel-wise comparison between synthesized CT and reference CT images. We do not expect this registration step to influence training, as training images were provided in a randomized unpaired way, making it unlikely that both an MR image and its registered corresponding CT image were simultaneously shown to the GAN. In addition, images were randomly cropped, which partially cancels the effects of rigid registration. Nevertheless, using images of the same patients in the MR set and the CT set may affect training. The synthesis networks could receive stronger feedback from the discriminator, which would occasionally see the corresponding reference image. In future work, we will extend the training set to investigate if we can similarly train the model with MR and CT images of *disjoint* patient sets.

References

1. Bahrami, K., Shi, F., Rekik, I., Shen, D.: Convolutional neural network for reconstruction of 7T-like Images from 3T MRI using appearance and anatomical features. In: Carneiro, G., Mateus, D., Peter, L., Bradley, A., Tavares, J.M.R.S., Belagiannis, V., Papa, J.P., Nascimento, J.C., Loog, M., Lu, Z., Cardoso, J.S., Cornebise, J. (eds.) LABELS/DLMIA -2016. LNCS, vol. 10008, pp. 39–47. Springer, Cham (2016). doi:10.1007/978-3-319-46976-8_5
2. Edmund, J.M., Nyholm, T.: A review of substitute CT generation for MRI-only radiation therapy. Radiat. Oncol. **12**(1), 28 (2017). doi:10.1186/s13014-016-0747
3. Goodfellow, I., Pouget-Abadie, J., Mirza, M., Xu, B., Warde-Farley, D., Ozair, S., Courville, A., Bengio, Y.: Generative adversarial nets. In: Advances in Neural Information Processing Systems, pp. 2672–2680 (2014)
4. Han, X.: MR-based synthetic CT generation using a deep convolutional neural network method. Med. Phys. **44**(4), 1408–1419 (2017)
5. Isola, P., Zhu, J.Y., Zhou, T., Efros, A.A.: Image-to-image translation with conditional adversarial networks. arXiv preprint (2016). arXiv:1611.07004
6. Johnson, J., Alahi, A., Fei-Fei, L.: Perceptual losses for real-time style transfer and super-resolution. In: Leibe, B., Matas, J., Sebe, N., Welling, M. (eds.) ECCV 2016. LNCS, vol. 9906, pp. 694–711. Springer, Cham (2016). doi:10.1007/978-3-319-46475-6_43
7. Kingma, D., Ba, J.: Adam: a method for stochastic optimization. In: ICLR (2015)
8. Nie, D., Cao, X., Gao, Y., Wang, L., Shen, D.: Estimating CT image from MRI data using 3D fully convolutional networks. In: Carneiro, G., Mateus, D., Peter, L., Bradley, A., Tavares, J.M.R.S., Belagiannis, V., Papa, J.P., Nascimento, J.C., Loog, M., Lu, Z., Cardoso, J.S., Cornebise, J. (eds.) LABELS/DLMIA -2016. LNCS, vol. 10008, pp. 170–178. Springer, Cham (2016). doi:10.1007/978-3-319-46976-8_18
9. Nie, D., Trullo, R., Petitjean, C., Ruan, S., Shen, D.: Medical image synthesis with context-aware generative adversarial networks. arXiv preprint (2016). arXiv:1612.05362
10. Wolterink, J.M., Leiner, T., Viergever, M.A., Isgum, I.: Generative adversarial networks for noise reduction in low-dose CT. IEEE Trans. Med. Imaging (2017). http://ieeexplore.ieee.org/document/7934380/
11. Yi, Z., Zhang, H., Gong, P.T., et al.: Dualgan: unsupervised dual learning for image-to-image translation. arXiv preprint (2017). arXiv:1704.02510
12. Zhu, J.Y., Park, T., Isola, P., Efros, A.A.: Unpaired image-to-image translation using cycle-consistent adversarial networks. arXiv preprint (2017). arXiv:1703.10593

Synthesizing CT from Ultrashort Echo-Time MR Images via Convolutional Neural Networks

Snehashis Roy[1(✉)], John A. Butman[2], and Dzung L. Pham[1]

[1] Center for Neuroscience and Regenerative Medicine,
Henry Jackson Foundation, Bethesda, USA
`snehashis.roy@nih.gov`
[2] Radiology and Imaging Sciences, Clinical Center,
National Institute of Health, Bethesda, USA

Abstract. With the increasing popularity of PET-MR scanners in clinical applications, synthesis of CT images from MR has been an important research topic. Accurate PET image reconstruction requires attenuation correction, which is based on the electron density of tissues and can be obtained from CT images. While CT measures electron density information for x-ray photons, MR images convey information about the magnetic properties of tissues. Therefore, with the advent of PET-MR systems, the attenuation coefficients need to be indirectly estimated from MR images. In this paper, we propose a fully convolutional neural network (CNN) based method to synthesize head CT from ultra-short echo-time (UTE) dual-echo MR images. Unlike traditional T_1-w images which do not have any bone signal, UTE images show some signal for bone, which makes it a good candidate for MR to CT synthesis. A notable advantage of our approach is that accurate results were achieved with a small training data set. Using an atlas of a single CT and dual-echo UTE pair, we train a deep neural network model to learn the transform of MR intensities to CT using patches. We compared our CNN based model with a state-of-the-art registration based as well as a Bayesian model based CT synthesis method, and showed that the proposed CNN model outperforms both of them. We also compared the proposed model when only T_1-w images are available instead of UTE, and show that UTE images produce better synthesis than using just T_1-w images.

1 Introduction

Accurate PET (positron emission tomography) image reconstruction requires correction for the attenuation of γ photons by tissue. The attenuation coefficients, called μ-maps, can be estimated from CT images, which are x-ray derived estimates of electron densities in tissues. Therefore PET-CT scanners are well suited for accurate PET reconstruction. In recent years, PET-MR scanners have become more popular in clinical settings. This is because of the fact that unlike

S. Roy—Support for this work included funding from the Department of Defense in the Center for Neuroscience and Regenerative Medicine.

© Springer International Publishing AG 2017
S.A. Tsaftaris et al. (Eds.): SASHIMI 2017, LNCS 10557, pp. 24–32, 2017.
DOI: 10.1007/978-3-319-68127-6_3

CT, MRI (magnetic resonance imaging) does not impart any radiation, and MR images have superior soft tissue contrast. However, an MR image voxel contains information about the magnetic properties of the tissues at that voxel, which has no direct relation to its electron density. Therefore synthesizing CT from MRI is an active area of research.

Several MR to CT synthesis methods for brain images have been proposed. Most of them can be categorized into two classes – segmentation based and atlas based. CT image intensities represent quantitative Hounsfeld Units (HU) and their standardized values are usually known for air, water, bone, and other brain tissues such as fat, muscle, grey matter (GM), white matter (WM), cerebrospinal fluid (CSF) etc. Segmentation based methods [2,13] first segment a T_1-w MR image of the whole head into multiple classes, such as bone, air, GM, and WM. Then each of the segmented classes are replaced with the mean HU for that tissue class, or the intensity at a voxel is obtained from the distribution of HU for the tissue type of that voxel.

Most segmentation based approaches rely on accurate multi-class segmentation of T_1-w images. However, traditional T_1-w images do not produce any signal for bone. As bone has the highest average HU compared to other soft tissues, accurate segmentation of bone is crucial for accurate PET reconstruction. Atlas based methods [6] can overcome this limitation via registration. An atlas usually consists of an MR and a co-registered CT pair. For a new subject, multiple atlas MR images can be deformably registered to the subject MR; then the deformed atlas CT images are combined using voxel based label fusion [3] to generate a synthetic subject CT. It has been shown that atlas based methods generally outperform segmentation based methods [6], because they do not need accurate segmentation of tissue classes, which can be difficult because it becomes indistinguishable from background, tissues with short T_1, and tissues whose signal may be suppressed, such as CSF.

One disadvantage of registration based methods is that a large number of atlases is needed for accurate synthesis. For example, 40 atlases were used in [3], leading to significantly high computational cost with such a large number of registrations. To alleviate this problem, atlas based patch matching methods have been proposed [17,19]. For a particular patch on a subject MR, relevant matching patches are found from atlas MR images. The atlases only need to be rigidly registered to the subject [19]. The matching atlas MR patches can either be found from a neighborhood of that subject MR patch [19], or from any location within the head [16,17]. Once the matching patches are found, their corresponding CT patches are averaged with weights based on the patch similarity to form a synthetic CT. The advantage of patch matching is that deformable registration is not needed, thereby decreasing the computational burden and increasing robustness to differences in the anatomical shape. These type of methods also require fewer atlases (e.g., 10 in [19] and 1 in [17]).

Recently, convolutional neural networks (CNN), or deep learning [12], has been extensively used in many medical imaging applications, such as lesions and tumor segmentation [9], brain segmentation, image synthesis, and skull stripping.

Unlike traditional machine learning algorithms, CNN models do not need hand-crafted features, and are therefore generalizable to a variety of problems. They can accommodate whole images or much larger patches (e.g., 17^3 in [9]) compared to smaller sized patches used in most patch based methods (e.g., 3^3 in [19]), thereby introducing better neighborhood information. A CNN model based on U-nets [15] has been recently proposed to synthesize CT from T_1-w images [5]. In this paper, we propose a synthesis method based on fully convolutional neural networks to generate CT images from dual-echo UTE images. We compare with two leading CT synthesis methods, one registration based [3] and one patch based [17], and show that our CNN model produces more accurate results compared to both of them. We also show that better synthesis can be obtained using UTE images rather than only T_1-w images.

2   Data Description

MR images were acquired on 7 patients on a 3T Siemens Biograph mMR. The MR acquisition includes T_1-w dual-echo UTE and MPRAGE images. The specifications of UTE images are as follows, image size $192 \times 192 \times 192$, resolution $1.56\,\mathrm{mm}^3$, repetition time $TR = 11.94\,\mathrm{s}$, echo time $TE = 70\,\mu\mathrm{s}$ and $2.46\,\mathrm{ms}$, flip angle $10°$. MPRAGE images were acquired with the following parameters, resolution $1.0\,\mathrm{mm}^3$, $TR = 2.53\,\mathrm{s}$, $TE = 3.03\,\mathrm{ms}$, flip angle $7°$. CT images were acquired on a Biograph 128 S PET/CT scanner with a tube voltage of 120 kVp, with dimensions of $512 \times 512 \times 149$, and resolution of $0.58 \times 0.58 \times 1.5\,\mathrm{mm}^3$. MPRAGE and CT were rigidly registered [1] to the second UTE image. All MR images were corrected for intensity inhomogeneities by N4 [20]. The necks were then removed from the MPRAGE images using FSL's `robustfov` [7]. Finally, to create a mask of the whole head, background noise was removed from the MPRAGE using Otsu's threshold [14]. UTE and CT images were masked by the headmask obtained from the corresponding MPRAGE. Note that the choice of MPRAGE to create the headmask is arbitrary, CT could also be used as well. The headmask was used for two purposes.

1. Training patches were obtained within the headmask, so that the center voxel of a patch contains either skull or brain.
2. Error metrics between synthetic CT and the original CT were computed only within the headmask.

3   Method

We propose a deep CNN model to synthesize CT from UTE images. Although theoretically the model can be used with whole images, we used patches due to memory limitations. Many CNN architectures have previously been proposed. In this paper, we adopt Inception blocks [18], that have been successfully used in many image classification and recognition problems in natural image processing

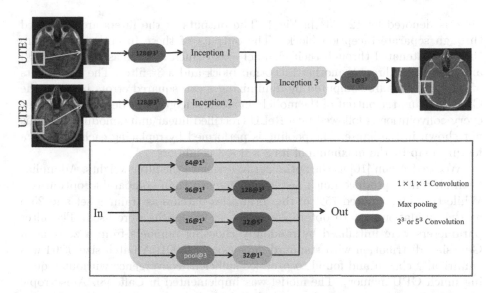

Fig. 1. The figure shows the proposed CNN model incorporating the Google Inception block [18], shown in inset. During training, patches from each of the dual-echo UTE images are first independently processed through two Inception blocks. Then their outputs are concatenated and again processed through another Inception block. Finally, the mean squared errors between the CT patch and the output of the third Inception block is minimized to train the parameters of the CNN. A convolution is written as $128@3^3$, indicating there are 128 filters of size $3 \times 3 \times 3$. The pooling layer is defined as `pool@3`, indicating maximum value within a $3 \times 3 \times 3$ region is used. Convolutions and pooling are done with stride 1. All convolutions are followed by ReLU, although for brevity, they are not shown here.

via GoogleNet. The rationale for using this architecture over U-net is discussed in Sect. 5. The proposed CNN architecture is shown in Fig. 1.

Convolutions and pooling are two basic building layers of any CNN model. Traditionally they are used in a linear manner, e.g. in text classification [11]. The primary innovation of the Inception module [18] was to use them in a parallel fashion. In an Inception module, there are two types of convolutions, one with traditional $n^3 (n > 1)$ filter banks, and one with 1^3 filter banks. It is noted that 1^3 filters are downsampling the number of channels. The 1^3 filters are used to separate initial number of channels (128) into multiple smaller sets (96, 16, and 64). Then the spatial correlation is extracted via $n^3 (n > 1)$ filters. The downsampling of channels and parallelization of layers reduce the total number of parameters to be estimated,which in turn introduces more non-linearity, thereby improving classification accuracy [4,18]. Note that the proposed model is fully convolutional, as we did not use a fully connected layer.

During training, $25 \times 25 \times 5$ patches around each voxel within the head-mask are extracted from the UTE images with stride 1. Then the patches from each UTE image are first convolved with 128 filters of size $3 \times 3 \times 3$. Such a filter is denoted by $128@3^3$ in Fig. 1. The outputs of the filters are processed through separate Inception blocks. The outputs of these Inception blocks are then concatenated through their channel axis (which is same as the filter axis) and processed through another Inception block and a 3^3 filter. The coefficients of all the filters are computed by minimizing mean squared errors between the CT patch and the output of the model via stochastic gradient descent. Note that every convolution is followed by a ReLU (rectified linear unit), module, which is not shown in the figure. The pooling is performed by replacing each voxel of a feature map by the maximum of its $3 \times 3 \times 3$ neighbors.

We used Adam [10] as the optimizer to estimate the filter weights. Adam has been shown to produce much faster convergence than comparable optimizers. While training, we used 75% of the total atlas patches as training set and 25% as the validation set. To obtain convergence, 25 epochs were used. The filter parameters were initialized by randomly choosing numbers from a zero-mean Gaussian distribution with standard deviation of 0.001. A batch size of 64 was empirically chosen and found to produce sufficient convergence without requiring much GPU memory. The model was implemented in Caffe [8]. Anisotropic $25 \times 25 \times 5$ patches were used because larger size isotropic patches requires more GPU memory, while the patch size was empirically estimated. To compensate for the fact that patches are anisotropic, the atlas was reoriented in three different orientations – axial, coronal, and sagittal. Training was performed separately for each oriented atlas to generate three models, one for each orientation. Then for a new subject, the models were applied on the corresponding reoriented versions of the subject, and then averaged to generate a mean synthetic CT. Training on a TITAN X GPU with 12 GB memory takes about 6 h. Synthesizing a CT image from a new subject takes about 30 s, where approximately 10 s is needed to predict one orientation. Although the training is performed using $25 \times 25 \times 5$ patches, the learnt models are able to predict a whole 2D slice of the image by applying the convolutions on every slice. Each of the three learnt models were used to predict every 2D slice of the image in each of the three orientations. Then the 3 predicted images were averaged to obtain the final synthetic CT.

4   Results

We compared our CNN based method to two algorithms, GENESIS [17] and intensity fusion [3]. GENESIS uses dual-echo UTE images and generates a synthetic CT based on another pair of UTE images as atlases. While GENESIS is a patch matching method which does not need any subject to atlas registration, the intensity fusion method (called "Fusion") registers atlas T_1-w images to a subject T_1-w image, and combines the registered atlas CT images based on locally normalized correlation. In our implementation of Fusion, the second echo of an UTE image pair was chosen as the subject image and was registered to the second echo UTE images of the atlases. The second echo was chosen for registration as its contrast closely matches the regular T_1-w contrast used in [3]. Similar to [5] which proposed a CNN model only using T_1-w images, we also compared the proposed model with both channels as the MPRAGE.

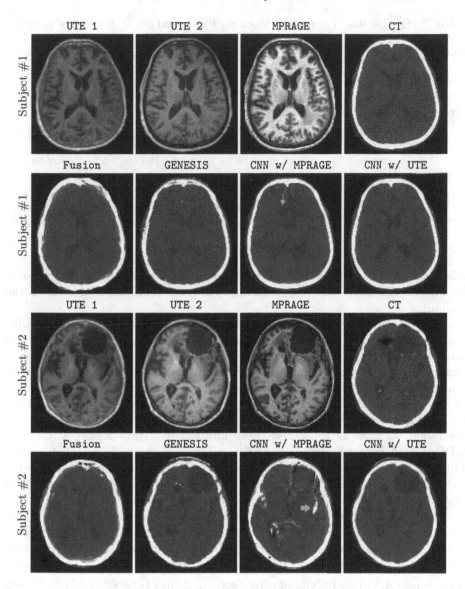

Fig. 2. Top two rows show UTE, MPRAGE, original, and synthetic CT images of a healthy volunteer. Bottom two rows show the same for a patient with a large lesion. Fusion [3] shows diffused bone in subject #1, while the CNN with MPRAGE shows some artifacts near ventricles (yellow arrow). Both GENESIS and the synthetic CT obtained with UTE can successfully reproduce the lesion (red arrow) for subject #2, with CNN synthesis showing less noise. (Color figure online)

One patient was arbitrarily chosen to be the "atlas" for both GENESIS and the proposed CNN model with both UTE and MPRAGE as inputs. The trained CNN models are applied to the other 6 subjects. Since Fusion requires multiple

Table 1. Quantitative comparison based on PSNR and linear correlation is shown for the competing methods on 6 subjects. Bold indicates largest value among the four synthetic CTs.

Metric	Method	Subject #					
		1	2	3	4	5	6
PSNR	Fusion	20.66	14.34	17.87	20.11	20.45	19.90
	GENESIS	18.89	16.28	17.20	17.96	21.52	21.17
	CNN w/MPRAGE	22.35	16.46	16.00	22.06	21.91	21.32
	CNN w/UTE	**23.40**	**18.76**	**19.78**	**23.49**	**23.54**	**22.54**
Correlation	Fusion	0.7377	0.6325	0.8097	0.7482	0.6807	0.6506
	GENESIS	0.5852	0.6800	0.7747	0.6277	0.6875	0.7132
	CNN w/MPRAGE	0.7851	0.6995	0.6867	0.8007	0.7160	0.7137
	CNN w/UTE	**0.8384**	**0.8457**	**0.8820**	**0.8634**	**0.8174**	**0.8017**

atlas registrations, the validation is computed in a leave-one-out manner only for Fusion. GENESIS was also trained on the same atlas and evaluated on the remaining 6.

Figure 2 shows examples of two subjects, one healthy volunteer and one with a large lesion in the left frontal cortex. For the healthy volunteer, all of the three methods perform similarly, while Fusion shows some diffused bone. It is because the deformable registrations can be erroneous, especially in presence of skull. CNN with MPRAGE shows some artifacts near ventricles (yellow arrow), while CNN with UTE images provide the closest representation to the original CT. For the subject with a brain lesion, Fusion can not successfully reproduce the lesion, as none of the atlases have any lesion in that region. CNN with MPRAGE shows artifacts where CSF is misrepresented as bone (blue arrow). This can be explained by the fact that both CSF and MPRAGE have low signal on MPRAGE. Synthetic CT from CNN with UTE shows the closest match to the CT, followed by GENESIS, which is noisier.

To quantitatively compare the competing methods, we used PSNR and linear correlation coefficient between the original CT and the synthetic CTs. PSNR is defined as a measure of mean squared error between original CT $\mathcal{A}$ and a synthetic CT $\mathcal{B}$ as, PSNR$= 10 \log_{10}(\frac{MAX_{\mathcal{A}}^2}{||\mathcal{A}-\mathcal{B}||^2})$, where $MAX_{\mathcal{A}}$ denotes the maximum value of the image $\mathcal{A}$. Larger PSNR indicates better matching between $\mathcal{A}$ and $\mathcal{B}$. Table 1 shows the PSNR and correlation for Fusion, GENESIS, the proposed CNN model with only MPRAGE and with dual-echo UTE images. The proposed model with UTE images produces the largest PSNR and correlation compared to both GENESIS and Fusion, as well as CNN with MPRAGE. A Wilcoxon signed rank test showed a p-value of 0.0312 comparing CNN with UTE with the other three for both PSNR and correlation, indicating significant improvement in CT synthesis. Note that we used only 6 atlases for our implementation of Fusion, although the original paper [3] recommended 40 atlases. Better performance would likely have been achieved with additional atlases. Nevertheless, the proposed model outperforms it with only one atlas.

5   Discussion

We have proposed a deep convolutional neural network model to synthesize CT from dual-echo UTE images. The advantage of a CNN model is that prediction of a new image takes less than a minute. This efficiency is especially useful in clinical scenarios when using PET-MR systems, where PET attenuation correction is immediately needed after MR acquisition. Another advantage of the CNN model is that no atlas registration is required. Although adding multiple atlases can increase the training time linearly, the prediction time ($\sim$30 s) is not affected by the number of atlases. This is significant in comparison with patch based [17, 19] and registration based approaches [3] ($\sim$1 h), where adding more atlases increases the prediction time linearly.

The primary limitation of the proposed, or in general, any CNN model is that it requires large amount of training data because the number of free parameters to estimate is usually large. In our case, by using only 3 Inception modules, the total number of free parameters are approximately 29,000. We used all patches inside the headmask which was about 500,000 for the 1.56 mm^3 UTE images. By adding more Inception modules, as done in GoogleNet [18], the number of free parameters grow exponentially, which needs more training data. An important advantage of the proposed model over the U-net in [5] is that only a single UTE image pair was used as atlas. Since we used patches instead of 2D slices [5, 15] for training, the number of training samples is not limited by the number of slices in an atlas. One atlas with 256 slices was used to generate 500,000 training samples, which was sufficient to produce better results than competing methods. In clinical applications, it can be difficult to obtain UTE and high resolution CT images for many subjects. Therefore using patches instead of slices give exponentially more training samples.

The patch size ($25 \times 25 \times 5$) is an important parameter of the model which was chosen empirically to make best practical use of the available GPU memory. Although CNN models do not need hand-crafted features, it was observed that using bigger patches usually increases accuracy. However, there lies a trade-off between patch size and available memory. Future work includes optimization of patch size and number of atlases, as well as exploring further CNN architectures.

References

1. Avants, B.B., et al.: A reproducible evaluation of ANTs similarity metric performance in brain image registration. Neuroimage **54**(3), 2033–2044 (2011)
2. Berker, Y., et al.: MRI-based attenuation correction for hybrid PET/MRI systems: a 4-class tissue segmentation technique using a combined ultrashort-echo-time/Dixon MRI sequence. J. Nucl. Med. **53**(5), 796–804 (2012)
3. Burgos, N., et al.: Attenuation correction synthesis for hybrid PET-MR scanners: application to brain studies. IEEE Trans. Med. Imaging **33**(12), 2332–2341 (2014)
4. Chollet, F.: Xception: deep learning with depthwise separable convolutions. In: arXiv preprint arXiv:1610.02357 (2016)
5. Han, X.: MR-based synthetic CT generation using a deep convolutional neural network method. Med. Phys. **44**(4), 1408–1419 (2017)

6. Hofmann, M., et al.: MRI-based attenuation correction for whole-body PET/MRI: quantitative evaluation of segmentation- and atlas-based methods. J. Nucl. Med. **52**(9), 1392–1399 (2011)
7. Jenkinson, M., et al.: FSL. NeuroImage **62**(2), 782–790 (2012)
8. Jia, Y., et al.: Caffe: convolutional architecture for fast feature embedding. In: 22nd ACM International Conference on Multimedia, pp. 675–678 (2014)
9. Kamnitsas, K., et al.: Efficient multi-scale 3D CNN with fully connected CRF for accurate brain lesion segmentation. Med. Image Anal. **36**, 61–78 (2017)
10. Kingma, D.P., Ba, J.: Adam: a method for stochastic optimization. In: International Conference on Learning Representations (ICLR) (2015)
11. LeCun, Y., Bottou, L., Bengio, Y.: Gradient-based learning applied to document recognition. Proc. IEEE **86**(11), 2278–2324 (1998)
12. LeCun, Y., et al.: Deep learning. Nature **521**(7553), 436–444 (2015)
13. Martinez-Moller, A., et al.: Tissue classification as a potential approach for attenuation correction in whole-body PET/MRI: evaluation with PET/CT data. J. Nucl. Med. **50**(4), 520–526 (2009)
14. Otsu, N.: A threshold selection method from gray-level histograms. IEEE Trans. Syst. Man Cybern. **9**(1), 62–66 (1979)
15. Ronneberger, O., Fischer, P., Brox, T.: U-Net: convolutional networks for biomedical image segmentation. In: Navab, N., Hornegger, J., Wells, W.M., Frangi, A.F. (eds.) MICCAI 2015. LNCS, vol. 9351, pp. 234–241. Springer, Cham (2015). doi:10.1007/978-3-319-24574-4_28
16. Roy, S., et al.: MR to CT registration of brains using image synthesis. In: Proceeding of SPIE Medical Imaging, vol. 9034, p. 903419 (2014)
17. Roy, S., et al.: PET attenuation correction using synthetic CT from ultrashort echo-time MR imaging. J. Nucl. Med. **55**(12), 2071–2077 (2014)
18. Szegedy, C., et al.: Going deeper with convolutions. In: International Conference on Computer Vision and Pattern Recognition (CVPR), pp. 1–9 (2015)
19. Torrado-Carvajal, A., et al.: Fast patch-based pseudo-CT synthesis from T1-weighted MR images for PET/MR attenuation correction in brain studies. J. Nucl. Med. **57**(1), 136–143 (2016)
20. Tustison, N.J., et al.: N4ITK: improved N3 bias correction. IEEE Trans. Med. Imaging **29**(6), 1310–1320 (2010)

A Supervoxel Based Random Forest Synthesis Framework for Bidirectional MR/CT Synthesis

Can Zhao[1]($\boxtimes$), Aaron Carass[1], Junghoon Lee[2],
Amod Jog[1], and Jerry L. Prince[1]

[1] Department of Electrical and Computer Engineering,
The Johns Hopkins University, Baltimore, MD 21218, USA
`czhao20@jhu.edu`
[2] Department of Radiation Oncology, The Johns Hopkins School of Medicine,
Baltimore, MD 21287, USA

Abstract. Synthesizing magnetic resonance (MR) and computed tomography (CT) images (from each other) has important implications for clinical neuroimaging. The MR to CT direction is critical for MRI-based radiotherapy planning and dose computation, whereas the CT to MR direction can provide an economic alternative to real MRI for image processing tasks. Additionally, synthesis in both directions can enhance MR/CT multi-modal image registration. Existing approaches have focused on synthesizing CT from MR. In this paper, we propose a multi-atlas based hybrid method to synthesize T1-weighted MR images from CT and CT images from T1-weighted MR images using a common framework. The task is carried out by: (a) computing a label field based on supervoxels for the subject image using joint label fusion; (b) correcting this result using a random forest classifier (RF-C); (c) spatial smoothing using a Markov random field; (d) synthesizing intensities using a set of RF regressors, one trained for each label. The algorithm is evaluated using a set of six registered CT and MR image pairs of the whole head.

Keywords: Synthesis · MR · CT · JLF · Segmentation · Random forest · MRF

1 Introduction

Synthesizing computed tomography (CT) images from magnetic resonance (MR) images has proven useful in positron emission tomography (PET)-MR image reconstruction [4,16] and in radiation therapy planning [5]. To overcome the lack of a strong MR signal in bone, one method [16] used specialized MR pulse sequences and another method [4] used multi-atlas registration with paired CT-MR atlas images. The synthesis of MR images from CT images is a new challenge that has not been reported until very recently [6,18]. Potential uses for this process include (1) intraoperative imaging where visualization of soft tissue from cone-beam CT could be enhanced by generation of a synthetic MR image and

© Springer International Publishing AG 2017
S.A. Tsaftaris et al. (Eds.): SASHIMI 2017, LNCS 10557, pp. 33–40, 2017.
DOI: 10.1007/978-3-319-68127-6_4

(2) in multi-modal registration where use of both modalities can improve the accuracy of registration [7,9]. The difficulty in CT-to-MR synthesis is the lack of a strong soft-tissue contrast in the source CT images. Given the duality that appears between these tasks, we have discovered a core organizing principle for bi-directional image synthesis and developed a new image synthesis approach.

To synthesize CT images from MR images, Burgos et al. [4] used multiple CT/MR atlas pairs, wherein the atlas MR images are deformably registered to the target MR image. The transformations are then applied to the atlas CT images and fused to form a single CT intensity. Although this approach can also be used to synthesize MR from CT, some degree of blurring can be expected due to the inaccuracies in registration due to poor soft-tissue contrast in the CT images. Machine-learning approaches that have been developed for image synthesis (cf. [8,15]) can also be used for synthesizing MR from CT; but image patches by themselves do not contain sufficient information to distinguish tissue types without additional information about the location of the patches.

Image segmentation has long been used for image synthesis [14]. If the tissue type and physical properties are known, then given the forward model of the imaging modality, the corresponding tissue intensity can be estimated. However, in our framework, segmented regions are used to provide *context* wherein synthesis can be carried out through a set of learned regressions that relate the intensities of the input modality to those of the target modality. We demonstrate synthesis in both directions, MR to CT and CT to MR, using our method.

2   Methods

Given a subject image of modality 1 (M1), denoted I^{M1}, our goal is to synthesize an image of modality 2 (M2), $\hat{I}^{M2}$. To achieve this goal, we have a multi-atlas set, $\mathcal{A} = \{(A_n^{M1}, A_n^{M2})| n = 1, ..., N\}$, which contains N pairs of co-registered images of M1 and M2. An example of an atlas pair, where M1 is CT and M2 is MR (T1-weighted) is depicted in Fig. 1(a). The two intensities in atlas image pairs are examples of possible synthetic values, when synthesizing in either direction. It is well known that this relationship is not a bijection; given an intensity in M1 there may be multiple corresponding intensities in M2. However, given a particular tissue (e.g., white matter) the relationship is less ambiguous. We carry out a segmentation on the atlas images that divides them into distinct regions characterized by different paired intensities. Paired intensities from these regions are then used to train separate regressors that predict one modality from the other given the tissue class.

We start with the atlas image set $\mathcal{A}$. Each pair of atlas images is processed with the following steps with the eventual goal of learning regressions that predict the target modality given the input modality. The first step is a supervoxel over-segmentation process using a 3D version of the *simple linear iterative clustering* (SLIC) method [1] wherein the intensity feature space comprises the M1 and M2 intensity pairs. A result of SLIC on two atlas pairs is shown in Fig. 1(b). Multichannel k-means and fuzzy k-means have been previously used for tissue

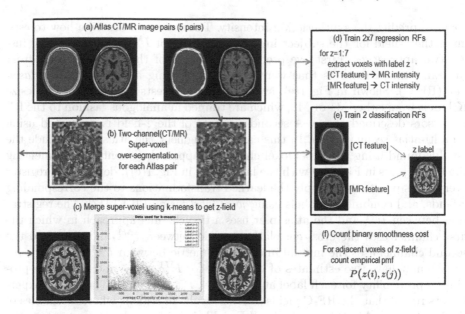

Fig. 1. (a) Two CT/MR atlas pairs; **(b)** result of SLIC over-segmentation; **(c)** k-means clustering of supervoxels yields a z-field image; **(d)** training of $2 \times K$ RF regressors; **(e)** RF-Cs trained to estimate z-fields from single modalities; and **(f)** computation of pairwise potentials for a MRF.

classification in neuroimaging [13]. However, it is difficult to obtain spatially contiguous regions using these simple methods. Super-voxel over-segmentation provides us with spatially contiguous regions that have homogeneous intensities.

We combine these homogeneous intensity regions by clustering them on the basis of their average supervoxel intensities taken jointly from both M1 and M2. These are clustered using the k-means clustering algorithm, which yields super-voxels that are labeled $z = 1, \ldots, K$. The voxels forming each supervoxel inherit the cluster label of the supervoxel and therefore yield an image of labels, which we call the z-field. Two examples of z-fields are shown in Fig. 1(c), where each label in the z-field is shown as a different color. A random selection of intensity pairs are plotted in the center of Fig. 1(c) (CT/MR on the horizontal/vertical axis), and colored by the z-field. These intensity pairs and their voxel-wise features, along with their labels provide the training data for regressors that predict the intensity of the target modality given the features of the input modality. Our features consist of $3 \times 3 \times 3$ image patches together with average image values in patches forming a constellation around the given voxel ("context features" similar to those in [2,10]). We need $2 \times K$ regressors, one each per modality and cluster. For each label z, we extract features from M1 images and pair them with corresponding M2 intensities. This acts as the training data set for a random forest (RF) regressor. The training step is depicted in Fig. 1(d).

Given the subject image I^{M1} and the corresponding z-field that labels its voxels, we can apply the corresponding regressor based on the z value at that voxel to predict the synthetic M2 intensity. Thus, we next describe how to estimate the z-field for the subject image. The z-field of I^{M1} is estimated by fusing two approaches. First, we predict an estimate of the z-field directly from the same image features that were noted above using a *random forest classifier* (RF-C). Shown in Fig. 1(e), are two random forests designed to synthesize K labels from either M1 or M2, which are trained in analogous fashion to the RF regressors described above. A second estimate of the z-field is generated using a multi-atlas segmentation. In this case, we augment the atlases to include the z-fields found using the supervoxel clustering approach (essentially augmenting the image pairs in Fig. 1(a) with the label fields in Fig. 1(c)), deformably register every atlas pair to I^{M1}, apply the learned transformations to the corresponding z-fields, and combine the labels using *joint label fusion* (JLF) [17]. The registration between I^{M1} and the atlas pair uses a two-channel approach in which the first channel uses the cross-correlation metric between I^{M1} and A^{M1} and the second channel uses the mutual information metric between I^{M1} and A^{M2}.

We now have two estimates of the z-field for I^{M1}, $\hat{z}_{\text{RF-C}}$ and $\hat{z}_{\text{JLF}}$, each provides a probability for each label at each voxel, $P_{\text{RF-C}}(z)$ and $P_{\text{JLF}}(z)$. Our experiments reveal that the RF-C yields inferior results in regions where intensities of the labels are ambiguous, while the JLF yields inferior results in areas where the registration is not accurate. We choose the label that maximizes the product of their probabilities at each voxel with a MRF spatial regularization.

Using a conventional MRF framework, we define the estimated z-field,

$$\hat{z} = \arg\min_{z(i)} \sum_i E_{\text{unary}}\big(z(i)\big) + \sum_{i,j} E_{\text{binary}}\big(z(i), z(j)\big), \tag{1}$$

where $E_{\text{unary}}\big(z(i)\big)$ is the unary potential for voxel i and $E_{\text{binary}}\big(z(i), z(j)\big)$ is the binary potential for adjacent (6-connected) voxels i and j. Since this energy will be used in a Gibbs distribution, the unary potential is defined as follows

$$E_{\text{unary}}\big(z(i)\big) = -\log P_{\text{RF-C}}\big(z(i)\big) - \log P_{\text{JLF}}\big(z(i)\big) \tag{2}$$

which yields the desired product of probabilities as the driving objective function for assigning labels to voxels.

Although the Potts model is often used in multi-label MRF models [11]—this is the model in which different labels have unity cost and similar labels have zero cost—we can exploit our atlas and its subsequent analysis to yield a cost function that is highly tailored to our application. Consider the z-fields produced by over-segmentation followed by k-means, as shown in Fig. 1(c), and consider adjacent voxels i and j. From the full collection of these images, we can compute the empirical joint probability mass function $P(z(i), z(j))$ for all adjacent voxels, as illustrated in Fig. 1(f). Some labels will almost never appear adjacent to each other and thus should be penalized heavily in the MRF we design. Accordingly, we define the binary potential as

$$E_{\text{binary}}\big(z(i), z(j)\big) = -\log P\big(z(i), z(j)\big) + \frac{1}{2}\big(\log P\left(z(i), z(i)\right) + \log P\left(z(j), z(j)\right)\big). \tag{3}$$

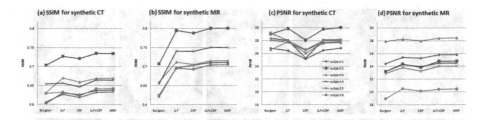

Fig. 2. Evaluation of synthesis result. The six colors are for six subjects.

When the labels are the same the cost is zero and when they are different, the cost increases according to their rarity of occurrence in the atlas. Given these definitions of unary and binary potentials (which is a semimetric), the estimated z-field is found by solving (1) using the α-β swap graph cut approach [3].

3   Experiments

MR images were obtained using Siemens Magnetom Espree 1.5 T scanner (Siemens Medical Solutions, Malvern, PA) and CT images were obtained using Philips Brilliance Big Bore scanner (Philips Medical Systems, Netherlands) under the routine clinical protocol from brain cancer patients treated by stereotactic-body radiation therapy (SBRT) or radiosurgery (SRS). Geometric distortions in MR images were then corrected using a 3D correction algorithm available in the Siemens Syngo console workstation. All MR images were then N4 corrected and normalized by aligning white matter peak identified by fuzzy C-means.

We applied our method to six subjects each having true CT and MR images to compare our results to. For algorithm comparison, we implemented [12] the intensity fusion method of Burgos et al. [4] using *structural similarity* (SSIM) as the local similarity measure instead of local normalized cross correlation (LNCC), which we refer to as Burgos+. Existing work on CT/MR synthesis [4] has focused on synthesizing CT from MR, so we can directly compare. Without a published method for synthesizing MR from CT, we simply applied Burgos+ in the reverse direction. To evaluate efficacy of synthesis, we computed SSIM and PSNR on the synthetic images with respect to the true images. The result is shown in Fig. 2. In addition to the comparison with Burgos+, we have shown how well modifications of our own algorithm perform. The "JLF" result uses only the z-field computed from JLF, the "RF-C" result uses only the z-field computed from RF-C, the "JLF+RF-C" result uses the product of the two z-field probabilities without MRF; and the "MRF" result is our proposed algorithm. We can see our method gives better synthetic MR in every respect, while the synthetic CT images are better than Burgos+ for SSIM and comparable for PSNR.

Figure 3 shows the estimated z-fields and final synthetic CT images for two subjects. It shows that our synthetic CT images have higher contrast and no blurry edges as compared to Burgos+, yet look somewhat artificial compared to

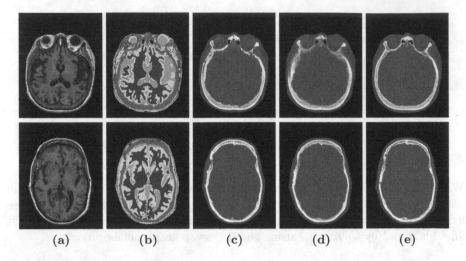

(a)   (b)   (c)   (d)   (e)

Fig. 3. Synthetic CT images: For two subjects, one in each row, we show the (a) input MR image, the (b) estimated z-field after MRF smoothing, the CT images generated by (c) our method, (d) Burgos+, and the (e) ground truth.

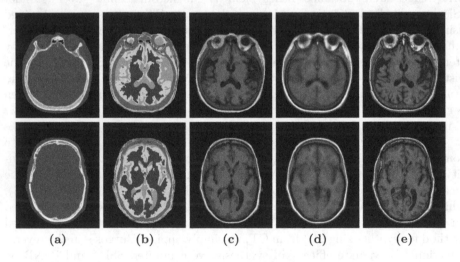

(a)   (b)   (c)   (d)   (e)

Fig. 4. Synthetic MR images: For two subjects, one in each row, we show the (a) input CT image, the (b) estimated z-field after MRF smoothing, the MR images generated by (c) our method, (d) Burgos+, and the (d) ground truth.

the truth. Figure 4 shows the estimated z-fields and final synthetic MR images for the same two subjects. It shows that our synthetic MR images also have high contrast and no blurry edges as compared to Burgos+. We notice in Fig. 4(e), the result from Burgos+ cannot synthesize the soft tissues correctly. This is because the result depends on the accuracy of registration between atlas image pairs and subject CT images, which is relatively low in areas of soft tissues. Our method

Table 1. Evaluation of registration results: Mean (and Std. Dev.) of MSE between reference MR and registered MR image; MI between target CT and registered MR image; p-value of paired-sample t-test for the MSE and MI of the two methods.

	MSE	MI
2 Channel CC	$2.746(\pm0.6492) \times 10^4$	$1.2314(\pm0.0746)$
Single Channel MI	$3.375(\pm0.6635) \times 10^4$	$1.2429(\pm0.1018)$
p-value over Single Channel MI	8.7637e–16	0.1962

is more robust to registration inaccuracies because we use a MRF to predict the z-field and the K random forests used in synthesis overlap in their intensity coverage to some extent.

To evaluate whether our synthesis method improves multi-modal registration, we carried out a multi-modal registration experiment between the CT image of one subject and the MR image of another subject. The conventional approach for multi-modal registration uses mutual information (MI) as a similarity metric. With synthetic images, multi-modal registration can be carried out using a two-channel mono-modal registration process [7,9]. In our case, for registration between Subject 1 and Subject 2, the first channel uses the original CT image of Subject 1 and the synthetic CT for Subject 2. The second channel uses the synthetic MR image of Subject 1 and the original MR image of Subject 2. The metric used in both channels is cross correlation (CC).

We used SyN deformable registration on 6 subjects yielding 30 pairs of registration experiments in all. The single MI registration and two-channel CC registration share the same parameters, including the number of iterations. As the true MR image is known, we compare the transformed MR image to the true MR image for each individual registration experiment. The difference between these two images is measured using both MSE and MI after either two-channel CC or single-channel MI (results are in Table 1). While the two images are not statistically different according to MI, the two-channel registration approach (which uses our synthetic images) is statistically better than the single-channel MI approach.

4   Conclusion

We have presented a bidirectional MR/CT synthesis method based on approximate tissue classification and image segmentation. The method synthesizes CT images from MR images with performance comparable to Burgos et al. [4] and is better than Burgos et al. [4] for synthesizing MR images from CT images. Our method reduces intensity ambiguity by estimating a z-field that is derived from both modalities and can be consistently created given just one modality as input.

Acknowledgments. This work was supported by NIH/NIBIB grant R01-EB017743.

References

1. Achanta, R., et al.: SLIC superpixels compared to state-of-the-art superpixel methods. IEEE Trans. Pattern Anal. Mach. Intell. **34**(11), 2274–2282 (2012)
2. Bai, W., et al.: Multi-atlas segmentation with augmented features for cardiac MR images. Med. Image Anal. **19**(1), 98–109 (2015)
3. Boykov, Y., et al.: Fast approximate energy minimization via graph cuts. IEEE Trans. Pattern Anal. Mach. Intell. **23**(11), 1222–1239 (2001)
4. Burgos, N., et al.: Attenuation correction synthesis for hybrid PET-MR scanners: application to brain studies. IEEE Trans. Med. Imaging **33**(12), 2332–2341 (2014)
5. Burgos, N., et al.: Robust CT synthesis for radiotherapy planning: application to the head and neck region. In: Navab, N., Hornegger, J., Wells, W.M., Frangi, A.F. (eds.) MICCAI 2015. LNCS, vol. 9350, pp. 476–484. Springer, Cham (2015). doi:10.1007/978-3-319-24571-3_57
6. Cao, X., et al.: Dual-core steered non-rigid registration for multi-modal images via bi-directional image synthesis. Med. Image Anal. **41**, 18–31 (2017)
7. Chen, M., et al.: Cross contrast multi-channel image registration using image synthesis for MR brain images. Med. Image Anal. **36**, 2–14 (2017)
8. Huynh, T., et al.: Estimating CT image from MRI data using structured random forest and auto-context model. IEEE Trans. Med. Imaging **35**(1), 174–183 (2016)
9. Iglesias, J.E., Konukoglu, E., Zikic, D., Glocker, B., Van Leemput, K., Fischl, B.: Is synthesizing MRI contrast useful for inter-modality analysis? In: Mori, K., Sakuma, I., Sato, Y., Barillot, C., Navab, N. (eds.) MICCAI 2013. LNCS, vol. 8149, pp. 631–638. Springer, Heidelberg (2013). doi:10.1007/978-3-642-40811-3_79
10. Jog, A., et al.: Random forest regression for magnetic resonance image synthesis. Med. Image Anal. **35**, 475–488 (2017)
11. Komodakis, N.: Image completion using global optimization. In: 2006 IEEE Computer Society Conference on Computer Vision and Pattern Recognition, vol. 1, pp. 442–452. IEEE (2006)
12. Lee, J., et al.: Multi-atlas-based CT synthesis from conventional MRI with patch-based refinement for MRI-based radiotherapy planning. In: SPIE Medical Imaging, pp. 101331I–101331I-6. International Society for Optics and Photonics (2017)
13. Pham, D.L., et al.: Current methods in medical image segmentation. Annu. Rev. Biomed. Eng. **2**(1), 315–337 (2000)
14. Riederer, S.J., et al.: Automated MR image synthesis: feasibility studies. Radiology **153**(1), 203–206 (1984)
15. Roy, S., et al.: Magnetic resonance image example-based contrast synthesis. IEEE Trans. Med. Imaging **32**(12), 2348–2363 (2013)
16. Roy, S., et al.: PET attenuation correction using synthetic CT from ultrashort echo-time MR imaging. J. Nucl. Med. **55**(12), 2071–2077 (2014)
17. Wang, H., et al.: Multi-atlas segmentation with joint label fusion. IEEE Trans. Pattern Anal. Mach. Intell. **35**(3), 611–623 (2013)
18. Zhao, C., et al.: Whole brain segmentation and labeling from CT using synthetic MR images. In: 8th International Workshop on Machine Learning in Medical Imaging. LNCS. Springer, Heidelberg (2017)

Region-Enhanced Joint Dictionary Learning for Cross-Modality Synthesis in Diffusion Tensor Imaging

Danyang Wang[✉], Yawen Huang[✉], and Alejandro F. Frangi

Department of Electronic and Electrical Engineering,
The University of Sheffield, Sheffield, UK
{dwang2,yhuang36,a.frangi}@sheffield.ac.uk

Abstract. Diffusion tensor imaging (DTI) has notoriously long acquisition times, and the sensitivity of the tensor computation often make this technique vulnerable to various interferences, for example, physiological motions, limited scanning time and patients with different medical conditions. In neuroimaging, studies usually involve different modalities. We considered the problem of inferring key information in DTI from other modalities. To address such a problem, several cross-modality image synthesis approaches have been proposed recently, in which the content of an image modality is reproduced based on those of another modality. However, these methods typically focus on two modalities of same complexity. In this work we propose a region-enhanced joint dictionary learning method that combines the region-specific information in a joint learning manner. The proposed method encodes intrinsic differences among different modalities, while the jointly learned dictionaries preserve common structures among them. Experimental results show that our approach has desirable properties on cross-modality image synthesis in diffusion tensor images.

Keywords: Dictionary learning · Cross-modality · Image synthesis · DTI

1 Introduction

Diffusion Tensor Imaging (DTI) offers a non-invasive *in vivo* imaging for mapping the diffusion of water molecules in the brain. The diffusion process is affected in different tissue microstructure, which makes evaluating the organizations and coherence of White Matter (WM) fiber tracts feasible. DTI is very sensitive to the motion of water molecules any physiological motions, e.g., subject motion, breathing and mechanical vibration, during the scanning time causes misalignment of the diffusion volumes. Particularly, the problem is further compounded in imaging patients with different medical conditions [1]. For example, patients with Parkinson's disease are difficult to stay stationary for even short time. In addition, long acquisition times of DTI scans is another limiting factor and also

© Springer International Publishing AG 2017
S.A. Tsaftaris et al. (Eds.): SASHIMI 2017, LNCS 10557, pp. 41–48, 2017.
DOI: 10.1007/978-3-319-68127-6_5

suffers from the effects on the suppression of physiological motions. Finally, in the most extreme case, acquiring a full battery of DTI also faces constraints associated with the patient's clinical state and severity of the disorder. DTI is not always performed, resulting in losing fundamental information needed for many later analyses, such as Electroencephalography (EEG) and Magnetic resonance elastography (MRE).

Cross-modality image synthesis is a classic task that seeks to synthesize the modality of a target image onto another input acquisition. The key challenges are to predict the structure and content of target modality image from the source image. It is of fundamental importance to many applications, including multi-modal registration, segmentation and atlas construction. Some early approaches rely on low-level statistics for image synthesis while using different ways to estimate the target image. For instance, histogram matching-based methods directly transfer one histogram into another by remapping the statistical profiles to obtain the target images. However, these methods often fail to capture modality-specific structures, especially with lacking the target modality images. Recently, several data-driven learning methods have shown exciting new perspectives for image synthesis. Jog et al. [2] introduced a nonlinear patch regression to synthesize T2-w contrasts from T1-w scans using the bagged ensemble of regression trees, which was later extended to synthesize the Fluid Attenuated Inversion Recovery (FLAIR) image from the corresponding T1-w, T2-w and PD-w images of the same subject obtaining better results in suppressing the artifacts on white matter lesions [6]. Roy et al. [3] trained two dictionaries where the input image is used to find the similar patches in a source modality dictionary and the corresponding target modality counterpart will be extracted in the target dictionary to generate the desirable modality data. A similar method had previously been used for image super-resolution [5]. Ye et al. [4] proposed a modality propagation method and proved that the proposed model can be derived from the generalization of label propagation strategy [7], and showed applications to arbitrary modality synthesis. The work of Nguyen et al. [8] is particularly relevant to deep learning, as they trained a location-sensitive deep network to integrate intensity feature and spatial information, more accurately synthesizing the results to the same problem posed by [4]. Huang et al. [9] improved the quality of cross-modality synthesis by imposing a graph Laplacian constraint in a joint learning framework. More recently, an simultaneous super-resolution and cross-modality synthesis approach [10] was proposed that up-converts a low-resolution result to a high-resolution one and synthesized the target modality synchronously.

In this paper, we propose a Region-Enhanced Joint Dictionary Learning (RJDL) method to synthesize the missing DT images from their T1-w scans by learning a region-enhanced joint dictionary based on the registered T1-w and DT images from training set. We consider the problem that white matter looks homogeneous in T1-weighted image, while it provides anisotropy information and orientations of fiber tracts in DTI. Although predicting the unknown fiber tracts in DTI from its T1-w acquisition is very ill-posed, we intend to overcome this problem by presenting a region-enhanced setting in a joint learning manner to improve the quality of our synthesis in WM region.

This paper is organized as follows. We explain the RJDL method in Sect. 2. Then we evaluate the proposed method on ADNI dataset and compare the synthesized results using RJDL and general joint dictionary learning in Sect. 3. Finally, Sect. 4 provides a conclusion and future work.

2   Method

2.1   Single Dictionary Learning

The basic idea of sparse coding is to construct a sparse representation of an input image $\mathbf{X}$ as a linear combination of a few dictionary elements, which chosen from an over-complete dictionary $\mathbf{D} \in \mathbb{R}^{n \times K}(n < K)$. Dictionary learning [11] aims to solve this optimization problem

$$\min_{\mathbf{D},\mathbf{A}} \|\mathbf{X} - \mathbf{DA}\|_2^2 + \lambda \|\mathbf{A}\|_0, \tag{1}$$

where $\mathbf{A} \in \mathbb{R}^{K \times N}$ is the sparse codes of $\mathbf{X} \in \mathbb{R}^{n \times N}$ with a few non-zero elements. $\|\mathbf{A}\|_0$ denotes the number of non-zero elements in the sparse codes and $\|\cdot\|_2$ is the Euclidean norm, and λ is a parameter to control the relationship between the reconstruction errors and sparsity penalty. Since the l_0-norm minimization problem is NP-hard (Nondeterministic Polynomial-time hard). An alternative solution was then proposed to solve this problem by replacing l_0-norm with its convex relaxation l_1-norm. The dictionary learning problem in Eq. (1) can be reformulated as

$$\min_{\mathbf{D},\mathbf{A}} \|\mathbf{X} - \mathbf{DA}\|_2^2 + \lambda \|\mathbf{A}\|_1, \tag{2}$$

Equation (2) is convex when $\mathbf{D}$ or $\mathbf{A}$ is fixed. When $\mathbf{D}$ is fixed, sparse code $\mathbf{A}$ can be solved as the Lasso problem; when $\mathbf{A}$ is fixed, $\mathbf{D}$ can be solved as a Quadratically Constrained Quadratic Programming (QCQP) problem. Updating $\mathbf{D}$ and $\mathbf{A}$ until the algorithm is guaranteed to convergence.

2.2   Region-Enhanced Setting

A major problem of cross-modality image synthesis between MRI and DTI is that white matter looks homogeneous in T1-w image, while uniform in corresponding DT images of the same subject. To efficiently leverage training data and consider that DT images provide more specific information in white matter than T1-w images, we propose a region-enhanced setting and integrate such region-specific information with joint dictionary learning. K-means clustering is applied to roughly cluster all samples to five major regions (white matter, gray matter, cerebrospinal fluid, ventricles and the others) according to the anatomical structures in brain of the DT images, and the corresponding T1-w patches are classified following the clustering results of DT images. We then recognize one of the cluster as the white matter region in visualization and preserve all elements of this cluster while randomly selecting a certain amount of instances from each of the remaining clusters.

2.3 Patch Normalization

Since different modality images have different intensity ranges, we must normalize all of them into a same range, i.e. $[-1, 1]$. The training data are firstly normalized by:

$$\delta = \max\{\|\mathbf{x}_i\|_2\}$$
$$\hat{\mathbf{x}}_i = \frac{\mathbf{x}_i}{\delta}. \tag{3}$$

where δ denotes the maximum norm value of all patches and $\{\mathbf{x}_i\}_{i=1}^{N}$ is the i-th element of $\mathbf{X}$.

2.4 Joint Dictionary Learning

Given a set of normalized T1-w image patches $\hat{\mathbf{X}} = \{\mathbf{x}_1, \mathbf{x}_2, \cdots, \mathbf{x}_N\}$ and the corresponding normalized DT images patches $\hat{\mathbf{Y}} = \{\mathbf{y}_1, \mathbf{y}_2, \cdots, \mathbf{y}_N\}$. In particular, each 4D DT image $\mathbf{Y}$ consists of six 3D tensor images denoted as $\mathbf{Y}_{xx}, \mathbf{Y}_{xy}, \mathbf{Y}_{xz}, \mathbf{Y}_{yy}, \mathbf{Y}_{yz}, \mathbf{Y}_{zz}$, and $\hat{\mathbf{Y}} = [\hat{\mathbf{Y}}_{xx}; \hat{\mathbf{Y}}_{xy}; \hat{\mathbf{Y}}_{xz}; \hat{\mathbf{Y}}_{yy}; \hat{\mathbf{Y}}_{yz}; \hat{\mathbf{Y}}_{zz}]$. We can train two separate dictionaries $\mathbf{D}^x$ and $\mathbf{D}^y$ using Eq. (2) for two sets of normalized training data:

$$\min_{\mathbf{D}^x, \mathbf{A}^x} \left\| \hat{\mathbf{X}} - \mathbf{D}^x \mathbf{A}^x \right\|_2^2 + \lambda \|\mathbf{A}^x\|_1$$
$$\min_{\mathbf{D}^y, \mathbf{A}^y} \left\| \hat{\mathbf{Y}} - \mathbf{D}^y \mathbf{A}^y \right\|_2^2 + \lambda \|\mathbf{A}^y\|_1. \tag{4}$$

where $\mathbf{D}^x$ and $\mathbf{A}^x$ are the learned dictionary and sparse codes of $\hat{\mathbf{X}}$, respectively. $\mathbf{D}^y$ and $\mathbf{A}^y$ denote the learned dictionary and sparse codes of $\hat{\mathbf{Y}}$, respectively. Unlike the single dictionary learning, Yang et al. [5] suggested to use a joint learning manner to train a pair of dictionaries $\mathbf{D}^x, \mathbf{D}^y$ from $\{\mathbf{X}, \mathbf{Y}\}$ to replace two independent learning. Based on such joint learning strategy, we assume that the co-registered patch pairs $\mathbf{x}_i, \mathbf{y}_{j_i}$ ($\mathbf{y}_{j_i}$ denotes the i-th patch from the j-th tensor matrix) possess the same intrinsic structure in a common space. This can be characterized by a jointly learned dictionary pair $\mathbf{D}^x, \mathbf{D}^y$ regarding the common sparse codes. This process can be written as this objective function:

$$\min_{\mathbf{D}^x, \mathbf{D}^y, \mathbf{A}} \left\| \hat{\mathbf{X}} - \mathbf{D}^x \mathbf{A} \right\|_2^2 + \left\| \hat{\mathbf{Y}} - \mathbf{D}^y \mathbf{A} \right\|_2^2 + \lambda \|\mathbf{A}\|_1, \tag{5}$$

where $\mathbf{A}$ represents the common sparse codes of $\hat{\mathbf{X}}$ and $\hat{\mathbf{Y}}$.

2.5 Objective Function

To improve the cross-modality image representation and facilitate specific region synthesis, we propose to learn a region-enhanced joint dictionary learning for cross-modality synthesis of DT images. The region-enhanced setting encodes region-specific features between images of different modalities in a particular region, while the joint learning strategy encodes the common features among different modalities to avoid multiple loss caused by several single dictionary learning.

We denote the common sub-coefficients associated with the c-th cluster of $\hat{\mathbf{X}}_c$ and $\hat{\mathbf{Y}}_c$ as $\mathbf{A}_c$, their corresponding sub-dictionaries as $\mathbf{D}_c^x$ and $\mathbf{D}_c^y$, where $c = 1, ..., C$. Mathematically we can express $\hat{\mathbf{Y}}_c$ using the joint learning manner as $\hat{\mathbf{Y}}_c \approx \mathbf{D}_c^y \mathbf{A}_c$. Instead of learning sub-dictionaries from all elements for each cluster, we only keep all data for a specific cluster while randomly extracting partial data for each of the reminding clusters. Ideally, more training data can provide richer information and yield better result for the stated specific region. We notice that the size of training data for such a specific region differs from other regions. To make sub-dictionaries to be incoherent, we follow the works [12,13] and add the constraints $\mathcal{R}^x(\mathbf{D}_c^x, \mathbf{D}_{-c}^x)$ and $\mathcal{R}^y(\mathbf{D}_c^y, \mathbf{D}_{-c}^y)$ to stabilize the learned sub-dictionary for each cluster, where $\mathbf{D}_{-c}^x = [\mathbf{D}_1^x, ..., \mathbf{D}_{c-1}^x, \mathbf{D}_{c+1}^x, ..., \mathbf{D}_C^x]$, $\mathbf{D}_{-c}^y = [\mathbf{D}_1^y, ..., \mathbf{D}_{c-1}^y, \mathbf{D}_{c+1}^y, ..., \mathbf{D}_C^y]$ are the sub-matrices by removing $\mathbf{D}_{-c}^x$ from $\mathbf{D}^x$ and $\mathbf{D}_{-c}^y$ from $\mathbf{D}^y$, respectively. The computation of the associated dictionaries and codes by minimizing the following objective function

$$\min_{\mathbf{D}_c^x, \mathbf{D}_c^y, \mathbf{A}_c} \sum_{c=1}^C (\left\| \hat{\mathbf{X}}_c - \mathbf{D}_c^x \mathbf{A}_c \right\|_F^2 + \left\| \hat{\mathbf{Y}}_c - \mathbf{D}_c^y \mathbf{A}_c \right\|_F^2$$
$$+ \lambda \left\| \mathbf{A}_c \right\|_1 + \gamma \left\| \mathbf{D}_c^{x^T} \mathbf{D}_{-c}^x \right\|_F^2 + \beta \left\| \mathbf{D}_c^{y^T} \mathbf{D}_{-c}^y \right\|_F^2). \tag{6}$$

where $\mathbf{A}_c$ denotes the common sparse codes for the c-th cluster data of $\hat{\mathbf{X}}_c$ and $\hat{\mathbf{Y}}_c$, $\|\cdot\|_F$ represents the Frobenius norm, γ and β represent the weight of incoherent terms for each modality respectively. Terms $\left\| \mathbf{D}_c^{x^T} \mathbf{D}_{-c}^x \right\|_F^2$ and $\left\| \mathbf{D}_c^{y^T} \mathbf{D}_{-c}^y \right\|_F^2$ are used to enforce sub-dictionaries of each modality to be incoherent.

2.6 Synthesis

Once the dictionaries $\mathbf{D}^x$ and $\mathbf{D}^y$ have learned from Eq. (6), we can calculate the sparse codes of T1-w test image regarding the same modality dictionary $\mathbf{D}^x$ using the conventional sparse representation in Eq. (2), denoted as

$$\mathbf{A}^t = \min_{\mathbf{D}^x, \mathbf{A}^t} \left\| \mathbf{X}^t - \mathbf{D}^x \mathbf{A}^t \right\|_2^2 + \lambda \left\| \mathbf{A}^t \right\|_1, \tag{7}$$

where $\mathbf{A}^t$ represents the sparse codes of the test image $\mathbf{X}^t$. We then utilize $\mathbf{A}^t$ as the common sparse codes and synthesize the target DT image of $\mathbf{X}^t$ by a linear combination of $\mathbf{X}^t$ and $\mathbf{D}^y$, obtaining

$$\mathbf{Y}^t = \mathbf{D}^y \mathbf{A}^t. \tag{8}$$

where $\mathbf{Y}^t$ is the synthesized results with six tensor images, i.e., $\mathbf{Y}_{xx}^t$, $\mathbf{Y}_{xy}^t$, $\mathbf{Y}_{xz}^t$, $\mathbf{Y}_{yy}^t$, $\mathbf{Y}_{yz}^t$, $\mathbf{Y}_{zz}^t$ included in a 4D matrix.

3   Experiments

3.1   Experimental Setting

In our experiments, we perform the proposed method RJDL on ADNI dataset[1] which allows us to observe healthy elders and Alzheimer's disease and early mild cognitive impairment. We randomly select 20 subjects of T1-w and Diffusion Weighted (DW) images from the whole dataset and use leave-one-out cross validation to evaluate the performance of our method. There are two pre-processing steps should be performed before the training stage, which is for guaranteeing the uniform sizes and co-registration of training pairs. First, Tortoise[2] is used to correcting the Diffusion Weighted (DW) images and estimation of the six DT images. Then, the registration of T1-w with DT images is implemented by 3D slicer[3]. We set the patch size as 55 pixels for both T1-w and DT images in all of our experiments, with overlap of 1 pixel between neighboring patches. Particularly, as mentioned in Sect. 2.3, the dictionaries for T1-w and DT images are trained from all patches in WM region/cluster and randomly extracted 100 patches in each non-WM cluster. This setting not only speeds up our algorithm at least four times, but also improves the quality of the synthesized images especially in white matter. Besides, we follows [5,9] and fix $\lambda = 0.15$ for sparsity regularization and the dictionary size as 1024 to balance the computation time and performance. The peak signal to noise ratio (PSNR) and structural similarity (SSIM) index [14] are used to measure errors.

Table 1. Quantitative evaluation on JDL vs. RJDL using the averaged PSNR and SSIM for total 20 subjects.

Avg.	JDL	RJDL
PSNR (dB)	30.98	**33.89**
SSIM	0.7963	**0.8458**

3.2   Results

We show a set of experimental results in Fig. 1 which compares the synthesized results using region-enhanced joint dictionary learning (RJDL) and joint dictionary learning (JDL). Compared to the general joint learning approach, our model trained for region-enhanced content synthesis does a very good job at synthesizing details of white matter region in DT images. Table 1 compares the performance of RJDL and JDL in terms of PSNR and SSIM, in which the average error measures (for all test images) are listed. It can be seen that our method achieved the highest PSNR and SSIM values for all of the test images, and generally outperformed JDL showed in the averaged synthesis results.

---

[1] ADNI dataset: http://adni.loni.usc.edu/.
[2] https://science.nichd.nih.gov/confluence/display/nihpd/TORTOISE.
[3] https://www.slicer.org/.

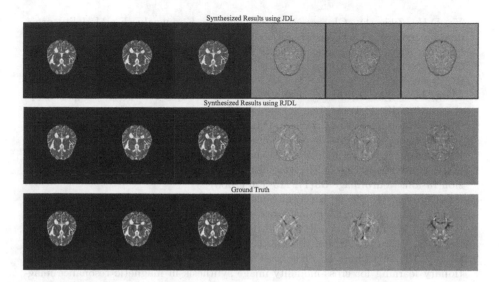

Fig. 1. The comparison of the synthesized results using JDL and RJDL regarding the corresponding ground truth images. The first line show the synthesized results using JDL, the second line gives the synthesized results using RJDL, and the third line presents the ground truth images. For each column, images from left to right are: $\mathbf{Y}_{xx}$, $\mathbf{Y}_{yy}$, $\mathbf{Y}_{zz}$, $\mathbf{Y}_{xy}$, $\mathbf{Y}_{xz}$, $\mathbf{Y}_{yz}$.

4   Conclusion

In this paper, we proposed a general and fast method to synthesize the unavailable DT images from the corresponding T1-w input. The proposed region-enhanced joint dictionary learning (RJDL) method shows its superior performance in accurate synthesis of DT image particularly in white matter region which do not appear in T1-w image. Our experimental results demonstrate the effectiveness of our RJDL, in which the quality of the synthesized results are better than the general joint learning approach. In future work, we will validate the proposed RJDL on the whole ADNI dataset and compare it with more state-of-the-art methods.

References

1. Aksoy, M., Forman, C., Straka, M., Skare, S., Holdsworth, S., Hornegger, J., Bammer, R.: Realtime optical motion correction for diffusion tensor imaging. Magn. Resonance Med. **66**(2), 366–378 (2011)
2. Jog, A., Roy, S., Carass, A., Prince, J.L.: Magnetic resonance image synthesis through patch regression. In: IEEE international Symposium on Biomedical Imaging, pp. 350–353 (2013)
3. Roy, S., Carass, A., Prince, J.L.: Magnetic resonance image example-based contrast synthesis. IEEE Trans. Med. Imaging **32**(12), 2348–2363 (2013)

4. Ye, D.H., Zikic, D., Glocker, B., Criminisi, A., Konukoglu, E.: Modality propagation: coherent synthesis of subject-specific scans with data-driven regularization. In: Mori, K., Sakuma, I., Sato, Y., Barillot, C., Navab, N. (eds.) MICCAI 2013. LNCS, vol. 8149, pp. 606–613. Springer, Heidelberg (2013). doi:10.1007/978-3-642-40811-3_76
5. Yang, J., Wright, J., Huang, T.S., Ma, Y.: Image super-resolution via sparse representation. IEEE Trans. Image Process. **19**(11), 2861–2873 (2010)
6. Jog, A., Carass, A., Roy, S., Pham, D.L., Prince, J.L.: MR image synthesis by contrast learning on neighborhood ensembles. Med. Image Anal. **24**(1), 63–76 (2015)
7. Heckemann, R.A., Hajnal, J.V., Aljabar, P., Rueckert, D., Hammers, A.: Automatic anatomical brain MRI segmentation combining label propagation and decision fusion. NeuroImage **33**(1), 115–126 (2006)
8. Van Nguyen, H., Zhou, K., Vemulapalli, R.: Cross-domain synthesis of medical images using efficient location-sensitive deep network. In: Navab, N., Hornegger, J., Wells, W.M., Frangi, A.F. (eds.) MICCAI 2015. LNCS, vol. 9349, pp. 677–684. Springer, Cham (2015). doi:10.1007/978-3-319-24553-9_83
9. Huang, Y., Beltrachini, L., Shao, L., Frangi, A.F.: Geometry regularized joint dictionary learning for cross-modality image synthesis in magnetic resonance imaging. In: Tsaftaris, S.A., Gooya, A., Frangi, A.F., Prince, J.L. (eds.) SASHIMI 2016. LNCS, vol. 9968, pp. 118–126. Springer, Cham (2016). doi:10.1007/978-3-319-46630-9_12
10. Huang, Y., Shao, L., Frangi, A.F.: Simultaneous super-resolution and cross-modality synthesis of 3D medical images using weakly-supervised joint convolutional sparse coding. In: The IEEE Conference on Computer Vision and Pattern Recognition, pp. 6067–6079 (2017)
11. Aharon, M., Elad, M., Bruckstein, A.: K-SVD: an algorithm for designing overcomplete dictionaries for sparse representation. IEEE Trans. Signal Process. **54**(11), 4311–4322 (2006)
12. Gao, S., Tsang, I.W.H., Ma, Y.: Learning category-specific dictionary and shared dictionary for fine-grained image categorization. IEEE Trans. Image Process. **23**(2), 623–634 (2014)
13. Ramirez, I., Sprechmann, P., Sapiro, G.: Classification and clustering via dictionary learning with structured incoherence and shared features. In: IEEE Conference on Computer Vision and Pattern Recognition, pp. 3501–3508 (2010)
14. Wang, Z., Bovik, A.C., Sheikh, H.R., Simoncelli, E.P.: Image quality assessment: from error visibility to structural similarity. IEEE Trans. Image Process. **13**(4), 600–612 (2004)

Virtual PET Images from CT Data Using Deep Convolutional Networks: Initial Results

Avi Ben-Cohen[1]([⊠]), Eyal Klang[2], Stephen P. Raskin[2],
Michal Marianne Amitai[2], and Hayit Greenspan[1]

[1] Medical Image Processing Laboratory, Department of Biomedical Engineering,
Faculty of Engineering, Tel Aviv University, 69978 Tel Aviv, Israel
avibenc@mail.tau.ac.il
[2] Sheba Medical Center, Diagnostic Imaging Department,
Abdominal Imaging Unit, Affiliated to Sackler School of Medicine,
Tel Aviv University, 52621 Tel Hashomer, Israel

Abstract. In this work we present a novel system for PET estimation using CT scans. We explore the use of fully convolutional networks (FCN) and conditional generative adversarial networks (GAN) to export PET data from CT data. Our dataset includes 25 pairs of PET and CT scans where 17 were used for training and 8 for testing. The system was tested for detection of malignant tumors in the liver region. Initial results look promising showing high detection performance with a TPR of 92.3% and FPR of 0.25 per case. Future work entails expansion of the current system to the entire body using a much larger dataset. Such a system can be used for tumor detection and drug treatment evaluation in a CT-only environment instead of the expansive and radioactive PET-CT scan.

Keywords: Deep learning · CT · PET · Image to image

1 Introduction

The combination of positron emission tomography (PET) and computerized tomography (CT) scanners have become a standard component of diagnosis and staging in oncology [7,13]. An increased accumulation of Fluoro-D-glucose (FDG), used in PET, relative to normal tissue is a useful marker for many cancers and can help in detection and localization of malignant tumors [7]. Additionally, PET/CT imaging is becoming an important evaluation tool for new drug therapies [14]. Although PET imaging has many advantages, it has a few disadvantages that make it a difficult treatment to receive. The radioactive component can be of risk for pregnant or breast feeding patients. Moreover, PET is a relatively new medical procedure that can be expensive. Hence, it is still not offered in the majority of medical centers in the world. The difficulty in providing PET imaging as part of a treatment raises the need for an alternative, less expensive, fast, and easy to use PET-like imaging. In this work we explore a virtual PET module that uses information from the CT data to estimate PET-like

© Springer International Publishing AG 2017
S.A. Tsaftaris et al. (Eds.): SASHIMI 2017, LNCS 10557, pp. 49–57, 2017.
DOI: 10.1007/978-3-319-68127-6_6

images with an emphasis on malignant lesions. To achieve the virtual PET we use advanced deep learning techniques with both fully convolutional networks and conditional adversarial networks as described in the following subsections.

1.1 Fully Convolutional Networks

In recent years, deep learning has become a dominant research topic in numerous fields. Specifically, Convolutional Neural Networks (CNN) have been used for many challenges in computer vision. CNN obtained outstanding performance on different tasks, such as visual object recognition, image classification, handwritten character recognition and more. Deep CNNs introduced by LeCun et al. [9], is a supervised learning model formed by multi-layer neural networks. CNNs are fully data-driven and can retrieve hierarchical features automatically by building high-level features from low-level ones, thus obviating the need to manually customize hand-crafted features. Previous works have shown the benefit of using a fully convolutional architecture for liver lesion detection and segmentation applications [2,3]. Fully convolutional networks (FCN) can take input of arbitrary size and produce correspondingly-sized output with efficient inference and learning. Unlike patch based methods, the loss function using this architecture is computed over the entire image. The network processes entire images instead of patches, which removes the need to select representative patches, eliminates redundant calculations where patches overlap, and therefore scales up more efficiently with image resolution. Moreover, there is a fusion of different scales by adding links that combine the final prediction layer with lower layers with finer strides.

1.2 Conditional Adversarial Networks

More recent works show the use of Generative Adversarial Networks (GANs) for image to image translation [6]. GANs are generative models that learn a mapping from random noise vector z to output image y [4]. In contrast, conditional GANs learn a mapping from observed image x and random noise vector z, to y. The generator G is trained to produce outputs that cannot be distinguished from "real" images by an adversarially trained discriminator, D, which is trained to do the best possible to detect the generator's "fakes". Figure 1 shows a diagram of this procedure.

In this study we explore FCN and conditional GAN for estimating PET-like images from CT volumes. The advantages of each method are used to create a realistic looking virtual PET images with specific attention to hepatic malignant tumors. To the best of our knowledge, this is the first work that explores CT to PET translation using deep learning.

2   Methods

Our framework includes three main modules: training module which includes the data preparation; testing module which accepts CT images as input and

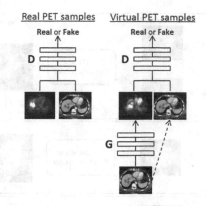

Fig. 1. Training a conditional GAN to predict PET images from CT images. The discriminator, D, learns to classify between real and synthesized pairs. The generator learns to fool the discriminator.

predicts the virtual PET image as output; blending module which blends the FCN and the conditional GANs output. The FCN and conditional GANs play the same role for training and testing. We explore and use both of them for the task of predicting PET-like images from CT images. Figure 2 shows a diagram of our general framework. Each module will be described in depth in the following subsections.

2.1 Training Data Preparation

The training input for the FCN or conditional GANs are two image types: source image (CT image) and target image (PET image) which should have identical size in our framework. Hence, the first step in preparing the data for training was aligning the PET scans with the CT scans using the given offset, pixel-spacing and slice-thickness of both scans. Secondly, we wanted to limit our PET values to a constrained range of interest. The standardized uptake value (SUV) is commonly used as a relative measure of FDG uptake [5] as in Eq. 1:

$$SUV = \frac{r}{a'/w} \tag{1}$$

where r is the radioactivity concentration [kBq/ml] measured by the PET scanner within a region of interest (ROI), a' is the decay-corrected amount of injected radiolabeled FDG [kBq], and w is the weight of the patient [g], which is used as a surrogate for a distribution volume of tracer. The maximum SUV (termed SUVmax) was used for quantitative evaluation [8].

Since the CT and PET scans include a large range of values, it makes it a difficult task for the network to learn the translation between these modalities and values range limitations were required. We used contrast adjustment, by clipping extreme values and scaling, to adjust the PET images into the SUV range of 0 to 20, this range includes most of the interesting SUV values to detect

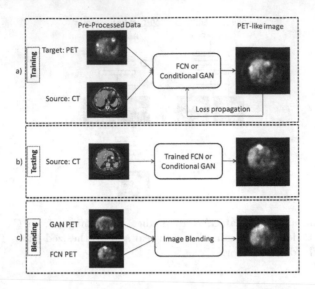

Fig. 2. The proposed virtual PET system.

tumor malignancies. Similarly, CT images were adjusted into −160 to 240 HU as this is, usually, a standard windowing used by the radiologists.

2.2   Fully Convolutional Network Architecture

In the following we describe the FCN used for both training and testing as in Fig. 2a and b. Our network architecture uses the VGG 16- layer net [12]. We decapitate the net by discarding the final classifier layer, and convert all fully connected layers to convolutions. We append a 1×1 convolution with channel dimension to predict the PET images. Upsampling is performed in-network for end-to-end learning by backpropagation from the pixelwise L_2 loss. The FCN-4s net was used as our network, which learned to combine coarse, high layer information with fine, low layer information as described in [11] with an additional skip connection by linking the Pool2 layer in a similar way to the linking of the Pool3 and Pool4 layers in Fig. 3.

2.3   Conditional GAN Architecture

Conditional GAN were used in a similar way described for the FCN in training and testing as in Fig. 2a and b. We adapt the conditional GAN architecture from the one presented in [6]. The generator in this architecture is "U-Net" based [10]. For the discriminator a "PatchGan" classifier [6] was used which only penalizes structure at the scale of image patches. Using a "PatchGan" the discriminator tries to classify if each 70×70 patch in the image is real or fake. Let C_k denote a Convolution-BatchNorm-ReLU layer with k filters and CD_k denotes a Convolution-BatchNorm-Dropout-ReLU layer with a dropout rate of 50%.

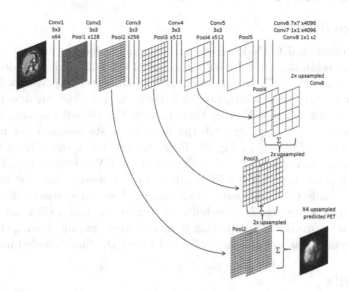

Fig. 3. FCN-4s architecture. Each convolution layer is illustrated by a straight line with the receptive field size and number of channels denoted above. The ReLU activation function and drop-out are not shown for brevity.

All convolutions are 4×4 spatial filters. Convolutions in the "U-Net" encoder, and in the discriminator (except of its last convolution layer), downsample by a factor of 2, whereas in the "U-Net" decoder they upsample by a factor of 2.

For the conditional GAN we used the following architecture:

– The discriminator: $C_{64} - C_{128} - C_{256} - C_{512} - C_1$.
– The "U-Net" encoder: $C_{64} - C_{128} - C_{256} - C_{512} - C_{512} - C_{512} - C_{512} - C_{512}$.
– The "U-Net" decoder: $CD_{512} - CD_{512} - CD_{512} - C_{512} - C_{512} - C_{256} - C_{128} - C_{64}$

The "U-Net" includes skip connections between each layer i in the encoder and layer $n - i$ in the decoder, where n is the total number of layers. The skip connections concatenate activations from layer i to layer $n - i$.

The "U-Net" generator is tasked to not only fool the discriminator but also to be similar to the real PET image in an L_2 sense, similar to the regression conducted in the FCN. For additional implementation details please refer to [6].

2.4   Loss Weights

Our study concentrates on the malignant tumors in PET scans. Malignant tumors are usually observed with high SUV values (>2.5) in PET scans. Hence, we used the SUV value in each pixel as a weight for the pixel-wise loss function. By this we allow the network to pay more attention to high SUV value even though most pixels include low values.

2.5   Image Blending

Since the conditional GAN learns to create realistic looking images its output was much more similar to real PET than that of the FCN that provided blurred images. However, the FCN based system had much better response to malignant tumors compared to the conditional GAN. Hence we used the advantages of each method to create a blended image that includes the realistic looking images of the conditional GAN together with the more accurate response for malignant tumors using the FCN as in Fig. 2c. First, we created a mask from the FCN output which includes regions with high predicted SUV values (>2.5). This mask marks the regions in which the FCN image will be used, where the rest of the image will include the conditional GAN image. A pyramid based blending was used [1]. Laplacian pyramids were built for each image and a Gaussian pyramid was built for the mask. The Laplacian pyramids were combined using the mask's Gaussian pyramid as weights and collapsed to get the final blended image.

3   Results

3.1   Dataset

The data used in this work includes CT scans with their corresponding PET scans from the Sheba Medical Center. The dataset contains 25 CT and PET pairs which we constrained to the region of the liver for our study. Not all PET/CT scans in our dataset included liver tumors. The training set included 17 PET/CT pairs and the testing was performed on 8 pairs.

3.2   Preliminary Results

The generated virtual PET image, per input CT scan, was visually evaluated by a radiologist. The virtual PET result was then compared to the real PET images by comparing tumor detection in the liver region. We define a detected tumor as a tumor that has SUVmax value greater than 2.5. Two evaluation measurements were computed, the true positive rate (TPR) and false positive rate (FPR) for each case as follows:

– *TPR*- Number of correctly detected tumors divided by the total number of tumors.
– *FPR*- Number of false positives per scan.

   The testing set included 8 CT scans with a total of 26 liver tumors. The corresponding PET scans were used as comparison with the predicted virtual PET. Our FCN and GANs based system successfully detected 24 out of 26 tumors (TPR of 92.3%) with only 2 false positives for all 8 scans (average FPR of 0.25).

   Figure 4 shows sample results obtained using the FCN, and FCN blended with the conditional GAN, compared to the real PET scan. False positive examples are shown in Fig. 5. In these cases, the FCN mistranslated hypodense regions in the liver to high SUV values.

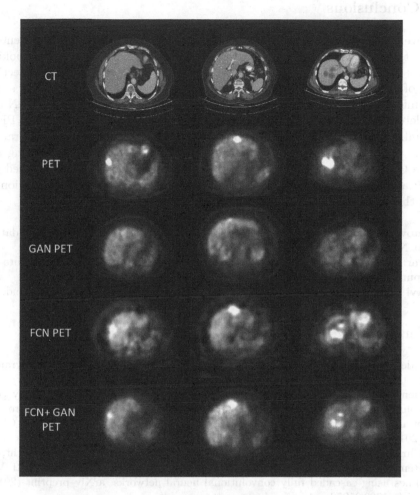

Fig. 4. Sample results of the predicted PET using FCN and conditional GAN compared to the real PET.

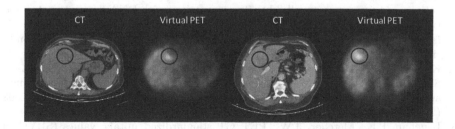

Fig. 5. False positive examples are marked with a black circle.

4   Conclusions

A novel system for PET estimation using only CT scans has been presented. Using the FCN with weighted regression loss together with the realistic looking images of the conditional GAN our virtual PET results look promising detecting most of the malignant tumors which were noted in the real PET with a very small amount of false positives. In comparison to the FCN the conditional GAN did not detect the tumors but obtained images which were very similar to real PET. A combination of both methods improved the FCN output blurred appearance. Future work entails obtaining a larger dataset with vast experiments using the entire CT and not just the liver region. The presented system can be used for many applications in which PET examination is needed such as evaluation of drug therapies and detection of malignant tumors.

Acknowledgment. This research was supported by the Israel Science Foundation (grant No. 1918/16).

Part of this work was funded by the INTEL Collaborative Research Institute for Computational Intelligence (ICRI-CI).

Avi Ben-Cohen's scholarship was funded by the Buchmann Scholarships Fund.

References

1. Adelson, E.H., Anderson, C.H., Bergen, J.R., Burt, P.J., Ogden, J.M.: Pyramid methods in image processing. RCA Eng. **29**(6), 33–41 (1984)
2. Ben-Cohen, A., Diamant, I., Klang, E., Amitai, M., Greenspan, H.: Fully convolutional network for liver segmentation and lesions detection. In: Carneiro, G., et al. (eds.) LABELS/DLMIA -2016. LNCS, vol. 10008, pp. 77–85. Springer, Cham (2016). doi:10.1007/978-3-319-46976-8_9
3. Christ, P.F., Ettlinger, F., Grün, F., Elshaera, M.E.A., Lipkova, J., Schlecht, S., Rempfler, M.: Automatic liver and tumor segmentation of CT and MRI Volumes using cascaded fully convolutional neural networks. arXiv preprint (2017). arXiv:1702.05970
4. Goodfellow, I., Pouget-Abadie, J., Mirza, M., Xu, B., Warde-Farley, D., Ozair, S., Bengio, Y.: Generative adversarial nets. In: Advances in Neural Information Processing Systems, pp. 2672–2680 (2014)
5. Higashi, K., Clavo, A.C., Wahl, R.L.: Does FDG uptake measure the proliferative activity of human cancer cells? In vitro comparison with DNA flow cytometry and tritiated thymidine uptake. J. Nuclear Med. **34**, 414 (1993)
6. Isola, P., Zhu, J.Y., Zhou, T., Efros, A.A.: Image-to-image translation with conditional adversarial networks. arXiv preprint (2016). arXiv:1611.07004
7. Kelloff, G.J., Hoffman, J.M., Johnson, B., Scher, H.I., Siegel, B.A., Cheng, E.Y., Shankar, L.: Progress and promise of FDG-PET imaging for cancer patient management and oncologic drug development. Clin. Cancer Res. **11**(8), 2785–2808 (2005)
8. Kinehan, P.E., Fletcher, J.W.: PET/CT standardized uptake values (SUVs) in clinical practice and assessing response to therapy. Semin. Ultrasound CT MRI **31**(6), 496–505 (2010)

9. LeCun, Y., Bottou, L., Bengio, Y., Haffner, P.: Gradient-based learning applied to document recognition. Proc. IEEE **86**(11), 2278–2324 (1998)
10. Ronneberger, O., Fischer, P., Brox, T.: U-Net: convolutional networks for biomedical image segmentation. In: Navab, N., Hornegger, J., Wells, W.M., Frangi, A.F. (eds.) MICCAI 2015. LNCS, vol. 9351, pp. 234–241. Springer, Cham (2015). doi:10.1007/978-3-319-24574-4_28
11. Shelhamer, E., Long, J., Darrell, T.: Fully convolutional networks for semantic segmentation. IEEE Trans. Pattern Anal. Mach. Intell. **39**, 640–651 (2016)
12. Simonyan, K., Zisserman, A.: Very deep convolutional networks for large-scale image recognition. arXiv preprint (2014). arXiv:1409.1556
13. Weber, W.A., Grosu, A.L., Czernin, J.: Technology insight: advances in molecular imaging and an appraisal of PET/CT scanning. Nature Clin. Pract. Oncol. **5**(3), 160–170 (2008)
14. Weber, W.A.: Assessing tumor response to therapy. J. Nucl. Med. **50**(Suppl 1), 1S–10S (2009)

Simulation and Processing Approaches
for Medical Imaging

Semi-supervised Assessment of Incomplete LV Coverage in Cardiac MRI Using Generative Adversarial Nets

Le Zhang$^{(\boxtimes)}$, Ali Gooya, and Alejandro F. Frangi

Department of Electronic and Electrical Engineering, Centre for Computational
Imaging and Simulation Technologies in Biomedicine (CISTIB),
University of Sheffield, Sheffield, UK
le.zhang@sheffield.ac.uk

Abstract. Cardiac magnetic resonance (CMR) images play a growing
role in diagnostic imaging of cardiovascular diseases. Ensuring full coverage of the Left Ventricle (LV) is a basic criteria of CMR image quality.
Complete LV coverage, from base to apex, precedes accurate cardiac volume and functional assessment. Incomplete coverage of the LV is identified through visual inspection, which is time-consuming and usually
done retrospectively in large imaging cohorts. In this paper, we propose a novel semi-supervised method to check the coverage of LV from
CMR images by using generative adversarial networks (GAN), we call
it Semi-Coupled-GANs (SCGANs). To identify missing basal and apical
slices in a CMR volume, a two-stage framework is proposed. First, the
SCGANs generate adversarial examples and extract high-level features
from the CMR images; then these image attributes are used to detect
missing basal and apical slices. We constructed extensive experiments to
validate the proposed method on UK Biobank with more than 6000 independent volumetric MR scans, which achieved high accuracy and robust
results for missing slice detection, comparable with those of state of the
art deep learning methods. The proposed method, in principle, can be
adapted to other CMR image data for LV coverage assessment.

1 Introduction

Left Ventricular (LV) cardiac anatomy and function are widely used for diagnosis and monitoring disease progression in cardiology and to assess the patient's
response to cardiac surgery and interventional procedures. Cardiac ultrasound
(US) and cardiac magnetic resonance (CMR) imaging are arguably the most
wide-spread techniques for clinical diagnostic imaging of the heart. For population imaging studies, however, CMR remains the modality of choice and provides
one-stop-shop access to cardiac anatomy and function non-invasively. The quantification of LV anatomy and function from large population imaging studies
or patient cohorts from large clinical trials requires automatic image quality
assessment and image analysis tools. A basic criteria for cardiac image quality
is LV coverage and detection of missing apical and basal CMR slices [7]. Due to

© Springer International Publishing AG 2017
S.A. Tsaftaris et al. (Eds.): SASHIMI 2017, LNCS 10557, pp. 61–68, 2017.
DOI: 10.1007/978-3-319-68127-6_7

rapid mechanical motion of the heart, breathing motion, and imperfect triggering, CMR can display incomplete LV coverage, which hampers quantitative LV characterization and diagnostic accuracy [12]. For example, missing basal slices has an important impact on LV volume calculation and several derived LV functional measures like ejection fraction and cardiac output. Even if scout images are acquired to center the LV in the field of view and minimize this problem, incomplete coverage can result at any points throughout the cardiac cycle due to patient breathing and cardiac motion. Automatic quality assessment is important in large-scale population imaging studies, where data is acquired across different imaging sites, from subjects with diverse constitutions, and with strict time constraints on scanner availability [4].

Few guidelines exist, clinical or otherwise, that objectively establish what constitutes a good medical image and a good CMR study [6]. To ensure consistent quantification of CMR data, automatic assessment of complete LV coverage is a first step. LV coverage is still assessed by visual inspection of CMR image sequences, which is subjective, repetitive, error prone, and time consuming [2]. Automatic coverage assessment must intervene and correct data acquisition soon, and/or discard promptly images with incomplete LV coverage whose analysis would otherwise impair any aggregated statistics over the cohort.

In medical imaging it is hard to have access to quality-labelled image databases due to the diversity of image characteristics, and their artifacts, of diverse anatomical locations and image modalities. Therefore, it is essential to devise techniques that do not require manual labelling of visual image quality. Image synthesis models provide a unique opportunity for performing unsupervised learning. These models build a rich prior over natural image statistics that can be leveraged by classifiers to improve predictions on datasets for which few labels exist [11]. Among them, generative adversarial networks (GAN) can synthesize adversarial examples, which increase the loss by a machine learning model [13]. Meanwhile, GAN can perform unsupervised learning by simply ignoring the component of the loss arising from class labels when a label is unavailable for a training image [5].

In this paper, we mainly focus on the analysis of short axis (SA) cine MRI. We aim to identify missing apical slices (MAS) and/or basal slices (MBS) in cardiac MRI volumes. In previous research, Le [14] used convolutional neural network (CNN) constructed on single-slice images and processed them sequentially. But this solution needs large amount of labelled data and lacks the ability to classify examples with perturbations correctly. In this paper, we exploit semi-coupled-GANs (SCGANs), a semi-supervised approach, for incomplete LV coverage detection. To alleviate the lack of sufficient numbers of CMR datasets with MBS or MAS, the proposed SCGANs use two generative models to synthesize adversarial examples. By learning adversarial examples, it improves not only robustness to adversarial examples, but also generalization performance for original examples. This work is the first work we know of to use adversarial examples to improve the robustness of an attribute learning model.

2   Methodology

We present a novel technique of LV coverage assessment for CMRI by using SCGANs. The motivation behind our proposed method is: In medical image quality assessment problems, we are always faced with a lack of quality-labelled data, especially images with artifacts. Several deep learning models cannot classify the examples with perturbation correctly. Our semi-supervised SCGANs is proposed by using adversarial examples as the outlying observations for discriminative model training. We generate adversarial samples by two generators separately, which confuse the discriminator into mistaking them for genuine images. After that, we obtain the robust attribute classifiers by learning both original data and synthetic data. Our proposed SCGANs represents a strategy to better handle the typical LV coverage assessment problem.

2.1   Generative Adversarial Learning

Recently, GAN [5] was proposed as a novel way for adversarial learning. It consists of a generative model and a discriminative model, both are realized as multilayer perceptrons [9]. The aim of the discriminator is to correctly classify the original examples and adversarial examples. By learning the adversarial examples, the network cannot only becomes robust to adversarial examples, but also generalization improves for unmodified examples. GAN does not need the label information when training the generator and then the discriminator can estimates the probability that a sample came from the original data rather than the generator.

We assume a probability distribution M, which is a black box relative to us. To realize how the black box works, we construct two 'adversarial' models: a generative model G that captures the data distribution, and a discriminative model D that estimates the probability that a sample from the training data rather than G. Both G and D could be a non-liner mapping function, such as a multi-layer perceptron. Our objective is to learn feature representation to handle a wide range of visual appearances in cardiac MRI and identify images with incomplete LV coverage. We regard adversarial examples as outlying observations regarding other samples in training data. The generative model constantly produce new adversarial samples and the discriminative model classify the positive and negative samples by learning the new produced adversarial samples constantly. Given a particular describable visual attribute - say 'MBS'. An outlier image is expected to be mapped to negative values, which indicates the absence of basal slice. This can happen for two reasons: (1) the image does not belong to the basal slice, (2) the image belongs to the adversarial examples. We consider them all as the outliers.

2.2   Semi-coupled GANs

Here we introduce our model based on the above discussion. Our model is illustrated in Fig. 1 designed as a semi-coupled-GANs for attribute learning. It consists of a pair of *Generators*− G_1 and G_2, which share a same discriminator. Each generator synthesizes the adversarial samples Y_1 and Y_2 for positive and negative data, respectively.

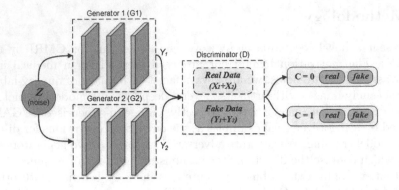

Fig. 1. The proposed semi-coupled-GANs framework.

Generative Models: We firstly feed the two generators G_1 and G_2 noise data z, G_1 and G_2 learn probability distribution from the original positive and negative images respectively, and generate the corresponding adversarial samples. Then, we give the adversarial data to discriminator D. Denote the distributions of $G_1(z)$ and $G_2(z)$ by p_{G_1} and p_{G_2}. Both G_1 and G_2 are realized as multilayer perceptions:

$$\begin{cases} G_1(z) = G_1^{(m_1)}(G_1^{(m_1-1)}(...G_1^{(2)}(G_1^{(1)}(z)))) \\ G_2(z) = G_2^{(m_2)}(G_2^{(m_2-1)}(...G_2^{(2)}(G_2^{(1)}(z)))) \end{cases} \tag{1}$$

where $G_1^{(i)}$ and $G_2^{(i)}$ are the ith layers of G_1 and G_2 and m_1 and m_2 are the numbers of layers in G_1 and G_2. In our training process, m_1 and m_2 need not to be the same. In traditional discriminative deep neural network, the feature information is extracted from low-level features in first layers to the high-level features in last layers. While, through multi-layer perceptron operations, our two generator models decode the information with an opposite flow direction from abstract concepts to more material details.

Discriminative Models: Every generated sample has a corresponding class label and the discriminator gives both a probability distribution over dataset and a probability distribution over the class labels. We put both the original samples and the adversarial samples into D for the discriminator training, D output multiple output values between 0 and 1. In this process, if the training samples x is the positive/or real data, the discriminant D ensures the output value is similar with the trained corresponding value, which represents the input data is the positive/or real, while output values close to 0 indicates the input data is the negative/or fake. The discriminant D equals a classifier with supervision situation, which returns to 1 or 0. Let D be the discriminative model given by:

$$D(x) = D^{(n)}(D^{(n-1)}(...D^{(2)}(D^{(1)}(x)))) \tag{2}$$

where $D^{(i)}$ is the ith layer of D and n is the number of layers. The discriminator maps each input image to a probability score which indicates the input is drawn from the positive data or the negative data. In this process, the first layer of the discriminative model extracts low-level features, while the last layer extracts high-level features.

Learning: The Semi-Coupled-GANs framework corresponds to a constrained minimax game given by

$$\max_{D} \min_{G_1,G_2} V(G_1, G_2, D) = E_{x \sim p_{x_{data}}}[\log D(x \mid y)] + E_{z \sim p_z}[\log(1 - D(G_1(z)))] \\ + E_{z \sim p_z}[\log(1 - D(G_2(z)))] \tag{3}$$

There are two terms in (3), each term has an independent generator but share a same discriminator. The two generative models synthesize a pair of adversarial samples for confusing the discriminative models. The discriminator gives both a probability distribution over image data and a probability distribution over the class labels, $D(x \mid y)$. Here, there are four kinds of samples for training the discriminator: the positive and negative samples from original images and their corresponding adversarial samples computed by two generators. The inputs discriminative model is data and corresponding labels. Similar to GAN, our SCGANs can be trained by back propagation with the alternating gradient update steps.

2.3 Quality Estimation

For a given cardiac volume, a dissimilarity score is computed for each representative visual attribute - MAS and MBS. Any visual attributes with a score below an optimal threshold is classified as an artifact. After computing the visual attributes, we could verify the cardiac MRI quality based on the corresponding attributes scores. Let $x_{target} = P_{MAS}(X_{target})$ and $y_{target} = P_{MBS}(X_{target})$ be the outputs of the discriminator. If the quality of target cardiac volume X_{target} is good, the values $P_{MAS}(X_{target})$ and $P_{MBS}(X_{target})$ from the target cardiac volume should be similar with the trained corresponding positive attribute values. We combine the output values so the verification classifier Q can make sense of the data. To address the problem, we use the concatenation of these tuples for both MAS and MBS attribute classifier outputs form the input to the verification classifier Q [8]. Finally, putting both terms together yields the tuples $q(S_{target})$:

$$q(S_{target}) = Q(<p_{MAS}, p_{MBS}>) \tag{4}$$

Training Q requires pairs of positive examples and negative examples. For the classification function, we use SVM with an RBF kernel for X, trained using libsvm [3] with the default parameters of $C = 1$ and $\gamma = 1/ndims$, where $ndims$ is the dimensionality of $<p_{MAS}, p_{MBS}>$.

3   Experiment and Related Analysis

Data specifications: In the UK Biobank (UKBB) dataset, we have 3400 subjects, each with 50 time points covering the heart from the base to apex. We use the endocardial contour as the main characteristic to identify the apical, middle and basal slices. For example, we can find the Left Ventricular Outflow Tract (LVOT) in the basal slice. In other slices, LVOT is nonexistant. As for the apical slice, we define it as the LV cavity is still visible at end-systole. Besides the basal slice and apical slice, we can consider the rest slices as the middle slices. To obtain the negative samples, we choose the middle slice as the negative samples for each attribute learning.

Experimental set-up: All experiments used TensorFlow [1] on GPUs. With all 50 time points consideration for each subject, we can obtain 17,0000 and regarded as the ground truth in our experiments. The architecture of the two generators G_1 and G_2 are consisted of several 'deconvolution' layers that transform the noise z and class c into an image [11]. We train the model architecture for generating images at 120×120 spatial resolutions. The discriminator D is a deep convolutional neural network with a Leaky ReLU nonlinearity [10]. In our experiment, 10-fold cross-validation method is used to evaluate the final performance of our attribute classifiers. To evaluate the classification algorithms, we use Accuracy, Precision Rate and Recall Rate defined as: $Accuracy = (TP + TN)/(TP + FP + TN + FN)$, $Precision\ Rate = TP/(TP + FP)$ and $Recall\ Rate = TP/(TP + FN)$. Where TP, TN, FP, and FN are the numbers of the true positive, true negative, false positive and false negative samples, respectively.

Performance and Discussion: We evaluate the quality of our semi-supervised representation learning algorithms by applying it as a feature extractor on supervised datasets. Table 1 shows the test performance on UK Biobank Dataset with the state-of-art deep learning methods. With supervised deep learning methods, 2D CNN, it achieved accuracies with 77.5% and 74.9%. Our SCGANs achieved performance with significant increase, 92.5% and 89.3% accuracies. This is despite the state of the art models having no ability to discriminate the adversarial samples, whereas our model requires to training the generative model to produce the adversarial examples and can correctly classify both unmodified and adversarial samples. It improves not only robustness to adversarial examples, but also generalization performance for original examples. Meanwhile, our SCGANs also achieved a comparable result with the 3D CNN, which indicates opportunity for future 3D image synthesis models.

Our attribute classifiers are trained using nine folds and then evaluated on the remaining fold, cycling through all ten folds. Receiver Operating Characteristic (ROC) curves are obtained by saving the classifier outputs for each test pair in all ten folds and then sliding a threshold over all output values to obtain different false positive/detection rates. In Fig. 2, we demonstrate the ROC curve to show that our adversarial training (SCGANs) method can achieve ideal results. These results reinforce that adversarial examples are powerful samples for attribute leaning. In Fig. 2 we can see our proposed method can correctly classify a few

Table 1. The accuracy, precision rate and recall rate between the state-of-art deep learning approaches and our method.

Method	Accuracy		Precision rate		Recall rate	
	MAS	MBS	MAS	MBS	MAS	MBS
2D CNN	77.5 ± 0.7%	74.9 ± 0.6%	82.6 ± 0.7%	74.9 ± 0.8%	87.7 ± 0.8%	87.8 ± 0.9%
3D CNN	93.1 ± 0.6%	91.8 ± 0.7%	90.1 ± 0.6%	87.3 ± 0.7%	89.9 ± 0.7%	93.3 ± 0.8%
Proposed method	92.5 ± 0.5%	89.3 ± 0.4%	87.6 ± 0.4%	89.1 ± 0.3%	90.5 ± 0.5%	91.7 ± 0.4%

challenging samples (True Positive) and adversarial samples (False Negative). Experimental results obtained confirm that adversarial training approach makes the model more robust to adversarial examples and generalization performance for original examples. Although the results show that the accuracy of the proposed method is slightly lower but comparable to that of 3D CNN, our SCGAN can reduce the computation cost, which is especially important in population imaging.

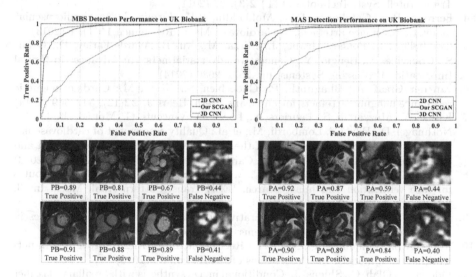

Fig. 2. MAS and MBS detection performance (Top) and sample test slices and their probability values (Bottom). 'PA' means the Probability value of being Apical slice; 'PB' means the Probability value of being Basal slice.

4 Conclusion

In this paper, we tackled the problem of defining missing apical and basal slices in large imaging databases. We illustrated the concept by proposing a SCGANs to CMR image studies from the UK Biobank pilot datasets. By training the classifier with the adversarial examples, our model can achieve a significant improvement in attribute representation. A well-trained attribute classifiers are performed on the candidates to corresponding categories. We also validated our model by comparing with traditional deep learning methods and applying them to UK Biobank data sets. The proposed model shows a high consistency with human perception and becomes superior compared to the state-of-the-art methods, showing its high potential. Our proposed semi-couple-GANs can also be easily applied and boost the results for other detection and segmentation tasks in medical image analysis.

References

1. Abadi, M., Agarwal, A., Barham, P., Brevdo, E., Chen, Z., Citro, C., Corrado, G.S., Davis, A., Dean, J., Devin, M., et al.: TensorFlow: large-scale machine learning on heterogeneous distributed systems. arXiv preprint (2016). arXiv:1603.04467
2. Attili, A.K., Schuster, A., Nagel, E., Reiber, J.H., van der Geest, R.J.: Quantification in cardiac MRI: advances in image acquisition and processing. Int. J. Cardiovasc. Imaging **26**(1), 27–40 (2010)
3. Chang, C.C., Lin, C.J.: LIBSVM: a library for support vector machines. ACM Trans. Intell. Syst. Technol. (TIST) **2**(3), 27 (2011)
4. Ferreira, P.F., Gatehouse, P.D., Mohiaddin, R.H., Firmin, D.N.: Cardiovascular magnetic resonance artefacts. J. Cardiovasc. Magn. Resonance **15**(1), 1 (2013)
5. Goodfellow, I., Pouget-Abadie, J., Mirza, M., Xu, B., Warde-Farley, D., Ozair, S., Courville, A., Bengio, Y.: Generative adversarial nets. In: Advances in Neural Information Processing Systems, pp. 2672–2680 (2014)
6. van der Graaf, A., Bhagirath, P., Ghoerbien, S., Götte, M.: Cardiac magnetic resonance imaging: artefacts for clinicians. Neth. Heart J. **22**(12), 542–549 (2014)
7. Klinke, V., Muzzarelli, S., Lauriers, N., Locca, D., Vincenti, G., Monney, P., Lu, C., Nothnagel, D., Pilz, G., Lombardi, M., et al.: Quality assessment of cardiovascular magnetic resonance in the setting of the european CMR registry: description and validation of standardized criteria. J. Cardiovasc. Magn. Resonance **15**(1), 1 (2013)
8. Kumar, N., Berg, A., Belhumeur, P.N., Nayar, S.: Describable visual attributes for face verification and image search. IEEE Trans. Pattern Anal. Mach. Intell. **33**(10), 1962–1977 (2011)
9. Liu, M.Y., Tuzel, O.: Coupled generative adversarial networks. In: Advances in Neural Information Processing Systems, pp. 469–477 (2016)
10. Maas, A.L., Hannun, A.Y., Ng, A.Y.: Rectifier nonlinearities improve neural network acoustic models. In: Proceedings of ICML, vol. 30 (2013)
11. Odena, A., Olah, C., Shlens, J.: Conditional image synthesis with auxiliary classifier gans. arXiv preprint (2016). arXiv:1610.09585
12. Pusey, E., Lufkin, R.B., Brown, R., Solomon, M.A., Stark, D.D., Tarr, R., Hanafee, W.: Magnetic resonance imaging artifacts: mechanism and clinical significance. Radiographics **6**(5), 891–911 (1986)
13. Szegedy, C., Zaremba, W., Sutskever, I., Bruna, J., Erhan, D., Goodfellow, I., Fergus, R.: Intriguing properties of neural networks. arXiv preprint (2013). arXiv:1312.6199
14. Zhang, L., Gooya, A., Dong, B., Hua, R., Petersen, S.E., Medrano-Gracia, P., Frangi, A.F.: Automated quality assessment of cardiac MR images using convolutional neural networks. In: Tsaftaris, S.A., Gooya, A., Frangi, A.F., Prince, J.L. (eds.) SASHIMI 2016. LNCS, vol. 9968, pp. 138–145. Springer, Cham (2016). doi:10.1007/978-3-319-46630-9_14

High Order Slice Interpolation
for Medical Images

Antal Horváth[1]([✉]), Simon Pezold[1], Matthias Weigel[1,2], Katrin Parmar[3],
and Philippe Cattin[1]

[1] Department of Biomedical Engineering,
University of Basel, Allschwil, Switzerland
`antal.horvath@unibas.ch`
[2] Radiological Physics, Clinics of Radiology,
University Hospital Basel, Basel, Switzerland
[3] Department of Neurology,
University Hospital Basel, Basel, Switzerland

Abstract. In this paper we introduce a high order object- and intensity-based method for slice interpolation. Similar structures along the slices are registered using a symmetric similarity measure to calculate displacement fields between neighboring slices. For the intensity-based and curvature-regularized registration no manual landmarks are needed but the structures between two subsequent slices have to be similar. The set of displacement fields is used to calculate a natural spline interpolation for structural motion that avoids kinks. Along every correspondence point trajectory, again high order intensity interpolating splines are calculated for gray values. We test our method on an artificial scenario and on real MR images. Leave-one-slice-out evaluations show that the proposed method improves the slice estimation compared to piecewise linear registration-based slice interpolation and cubic interpolation.

Keywords: Slice interpolation · Image registration · Splines

1 Introduction

Medical images often have anisotropic resolution. For example, in magnetic resonance (MR) images the in-plane resolution is often higher than the through-plane resolution. Reslicing and upsampling are standard preprocessing steps when dealing with such data. This motivates the search for slice interpolating methods to increase the resolution between the slices. Standard intensity interpolations such as *nearest neighbor*, *linear*, or *cubic* interpolations are well established. By using such intensity interpolations between two slices with different structure we would calculate linear combinations of intensities of points that do not belong together, see Fig. 2 row 3 in the red box. Therefore it is better to interpolate the object structure and position, which involves registration techniques to find correspondences. Morphing images is often done using manual landmarks, but since putting landmarks manually would be tedious, an automatic registration is

© Springer International Publishing AG 2017
S.A. Tsaftaris et al. (Eds.): SASHIMI 2017, LNCS 10557, pp. 69–78, 2017.
DOI: 10.1007/978-3-319-68127-6_8

advantageous. Grevera et al. [4] present a first comparison of slice interpolation methods that use correspondence points. In general, to guarantee meaningful slice interpolations, the structures of two subsequent slices have to be similar and the registration approach has to find an appropriate displacement field. Registration-based slice interpolation is an important field of research. Penney et al. [7] use a nonrigid registration algorithm with a spatial B-spline basis [8] but linear interpolation along the displacement field. Frakes et al. [3] use a modified version of control grid interpolation and a cubic interpolator for the displacement fields. Leng et al. [6] use a multi-resolution registration method and linear intensity interpolation along Catmull-Rom spline interpolated displacement fields.

Baghaie et al. [1] introduce a method with a symmetric similarity measure and curvature regularization

$$\underset{v:\Omega\to\mathbb{R}^2}{\operatorname{argmin}} \frac{1}{2} \int_{\Omega} [I_1(\mathbf{x} - v(\mathbf{x})/2) - I_2(\mathbf{x} + v(\mathbf{x})/2)]^2 + \lambda \left((\Delta v_x(\mathbf{x}))^2 + (\Delta v_y(\mathbf{x}))^2\right) \, d\mathbf{x},$$

(1)

where they look for a displacement field v by minimizing the intensity differences between the simultaneously displaced images and the bending of the resulting displacement field. The two images I_1 and I_2 share the common intrinsic image domain $\Omega \subset \mathbb{R}^2$ and v_x and v_y are the displacement field components in x and y direction. Using a symmetric similarity has the advantage that both the "reference" and "target" can be warped in a more symmetric way. After minimizing energy (1), they can interpolate an image $1/2 I_1(\mathbf{x} - v(\mathbf{x})/2) + 1/2 I_2(\mathbf{x} + v(\mathbf{x})/2)$ in the middle of I_1 and I_2 through linear intensity interpolation at the automatically registered and transformed correspondence points.

As an analytical property the zero level set of the curvature regularization contains harmonic functions and among them affine transformations [2]. This means that during minimization processes affine transformations are preferred as long as possible, as can be nicely seen in an example in [2, Fig. 2]. Moreover, the gradient descent steps with the curvature regularization can be iterated efficiently with a stable, implicit finite difference scheme.

Stacking together these linear interpolations between many neighboring slices results in a piecewise linear interpolation. At the stitching points, kinks may appear, which could be smoothed out using a higher order interpolation; see Fig. 1, left.

In this paper we derive a method that interpolates a whole stack of images through both object and intensity interpolation. Given the point correspondences between the slices, it calculates spline trajectories for all the correspondences and along these trajectories spline interpolations for the gray values; see Fig. 1, right. To find the correspondences between the slices we use the slice registration proposed in [1], but the proposed method can easily be adapted to other distance measures. Our contribution lies in solving the problem of combining higher order interpolations of structure motion and intensity. We describe the approach and the algorithm in Sect. 2, we test the proposed method on a test scenario and on real 3D images in Sect. 3, and we conclude in Sect. 4.

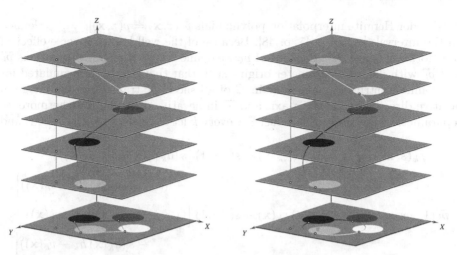

Fig. 1. Registration-based slice interpolation schemes: piecewise linear *(left)* vs. smooth interpolation *(right)*, with their projections on the x-y-planes *(bottom)*. In both interpolations on the left and right, two exemplary correspondence curves are shown: correspondences of points in a flat region and correspondences of a boundary pixel of the circling ellipse. To get a full interpolation, for all pixels in the slices such correspondence curves are established. The proposed method optimizes over the whole z range for a smooth interpolation, similar as in the right scheme, avoiding kinks on the correspondence curves at the given slice positions.

2 Method

Let $(I_k)_{k=1,\ldots,P}$ be an ordered stack of P similar 2D images in $\mathbb{R}^{M \times N}$, i.e. the slices of a volumetric image or the frames of a movie. Assume slices I_k lie parallel to the x-y-plane and their positions $z_k \in \mathbb{R}$ along the z-axis are given with $z_k < z_{k+1}$. Our task is to interpolate a new slice at any distance between two subsequent slices or to refine the slice distances $h_k = z_{k+1} - z_k$ by a factor $R \in \mathbb{N}$.

Given an image distance measure $\mathcal{D}$ and a displacement field regularization $\mathcal{R}$, we minimize the summed up registration energies of all the neighboring image pairs at specific registration evaluation points $\mathcal{S}$ along the z-axis:

$$\underset{\mathbf{v}=\{v_k:\Omega\to\mathbb{R}^2\}_{k=1}^{P-1}}{\operatorname{argmin}} \sum_{k=1}^{P-1}\sum_{s\in\mathcal{S}} \mathcal{D}\left[I_k \circ \overrightarrow{p_k}(s), I_{k+1} \circ \overleftarrow{p_k}(1-s)\right] + \lambda\,\mathcal{R}(\mathbf{v}_k). \quad (2)$$

Similar to [1], we use sum of squared distances for $\mathcal{D}$ and curvature regularization for $\mathcal{R}$ [2] but add the evaluation points $\mathcal{S} = \{0, 1/2, 1\}$. To clarify the notation, the intensity of the transformed images $I \circ p(z)$ at point $\mathbf{x}$ in the intrinsic image domain Ω can be read out by $I(p(z,\mathbf{x}))$, whereas the transformations $\overrightarrow{p_k}(s,\mathbf{x})$ and $\overleftarrow{p_k}(1-s,\mathbf{x})$ are defined as follows: For each point $\mathbf{x}$ we interpolate a trajectory $p(z,\mathbf{x})$ for $z \in [z_1, z_P]$ along the slices. With the displacement fields v_k, which give correspondences for subsequent slices, we construct a natural spline with the third order Hermite interpolation polynomials $p_k(z, \mathbf{x}) = p(z, \mathbf{x})|_{[z_k, z_{k+1}]}$ defined on the intervals $[z_k, z_{k+1}]$ [5, p. 48]. Because of the well known inverse effect of transforming image domains, out of p_k we define two special transformations $\overrightarrow{p_k}$ and $\overleftarrow{p_k}$ with different parameter origins such that they are both formulated for the common intrinsic image domain Ω of all slices: $\overrightarrow{p_k}$ transforms the image in positive direction along the z-axis and $\overleftarrow{p_k}$ in negative direction. Furthermore we reparametrize the transformations. For every k let $z = z_k + s\, h_k$ with $s \in [0, 1]$ and

$$\overrightarrow{p_k}(s, \mathbf{x}) = \mathbf{x} \quad - s\, v_k(\mathbf{x}) - s(s-1) \Big[s\, (a_{k+1}(\mathbf{x})\, h_k - v_k(\mathbf{x})) +$$
$$+ (s-1)\, (a_k(\mathbf{x})\, h_k - v_k(\mathbf{x})) \Big],$$

$$\overleftarrow{p_k}(1-s, \mathbf{x}) = \mathbf{x} \quad + (1-s)\, v_k(\mathbf{x}) - s(s-1) \Big[(1-s)\, (a_{k+1}(\mathbf{x})\, h_k - v_k(\mathbf{x})) +$$
$$- s\, (a_k(\mathbf{x})\, h_k - v_k(\mathbf{x})) \Big].$$

For using piecewise polynomial Lagrange interpolation of degree three, four supporting points, or more abstractly, four degrees of freedom have to be set on each interval $[z_k, z_{k+1}]$. Between the obvious supporting points $p_k(z_k, \mathbf{x}) = \mathbf{x}$ and $p_k(z_{k+1}, \mathbf{x}) = \mathbf{x} + v_k(\mathbf{x})$ the remaining two are placed exactly at the same spots z_k and z_{k+1} [5]. At the positions where two supporting points are now on top of each other, Hermite interpolation can be used to calculate the derivatives $a_k = p'(z_k)$ and $a_{k+1} = p'(z_{k+1})$. They define the other two degrees of freedom. The slopes a_k can be calculated through a nicely conditioned tridiagonal linear equation system of size $P \times P$ by incorporating smoothness conditions of the trajectory interpolation p. For the third order spline to be two times differentiable, the first and second derivatives at the stitching positions of the neighboring interpolation polynomials are set to be equivalent: $p_k'(z_{k+1}) = p_{k+1}'(z_{k+1})$, $p_k''(z_{k+1}) = p_{k+1}''(z_{k+1})$. This way, along each correspondence point trajectory, the spline interpolator minimizes the bending energy $\int_{z_1}^{z_P} (p''(z))^2 \, dz$ among all two times differentiable interpolators [5]. Adding the natural spline condition $p''(z_1) = p''(z_P) = 0$ defines all the degrees of freedom for the splines. For every $\mathbf{x} \in \Omega$, the optimal first derivatives $a(\mathbf{x}) = (a_k(\mathbf{x}))_{k=1,...,P} = ((a_{kx}(\mathbf{x}), a_{ky}(\mathbf{x})))_{k=1,...,P}$ in x and y direction now can be calculated through solving the $2 \cdot M \cdot N$ linear systems $A\, a_{.x}(\mathbf{x}) = d_{.x}(\mathbf{x})$ and $A\, a_{.y}(\mathbf{x}) = d_{.y}(\mathbf{x})$ of size $P \times P$, where

$$A = \begin{pmatrix} 2 & 1 & 0 & \cdots & & & 0 \\ \frac{1}{h_1} & 2\left(\frac{1}{h_1}+\frac{1}{h_2}\right) & \frac{1}{h_2} & 0 & & \cdots & 0 \\ 0 & & \ddots & & & & \vdots \\ \vdots & & & & & & \\ & & & \frac{1}{h_{P-2}} & 2\left(\frac{1}{h_{P-2}}+\frac{1}{h_{P-1}}\right) & \frac{1}{h_{P-1}} \\ 0 & \cdots & & & 0 & 1 & 2 \end{pmatrix},$$

$$d_1(\mathbf{x}) = 3\frac{v_1(\mathbf{x})}{h_1},$$
$$d_k(\mathbf{x}) = 3\left(\frac{v_{k-1}(\mathbf{x})}{h_{k-1}} + \frac{v_k(\mathbf{x})}{h_k}\right),$$
$$d_P(\mathbf{x}) = 3\frac{v_{P-1}(\mathbf{x})}{h_{P-1}}.$$

$$(3)$$

These systems can efficiently be solved by exploiting the structure of the invertible tridiagonal matrix A. After a Cholesky decomposition $A = LL^T$, the systems $A\, a = d$ can be rewritten by $L\, e = d$ and $L^T a = e$. The lower triangular matrix

---

Algorithm 1. Proposed Slice Interpolation Algorithm

Data: slices $I \in \mathbb{R}^{M \times N \times P}$, slice distances $h \in \mathbb{R}^{P-1}$, refinement factor R
Result: interpolated slices $I^{\text{interp}} \in \mathbb{R}^{M \times N \times ((P-1)R+1)}$
Set up the spline matrix $A \in \mathbb{R}^{P \times P}$ and calculate Cholesky decomp $A = LL^T$.
Calculate $D \in \mathbb{R}^{M \times N}$, $D_{ij} = 1 + \tau \lambda \left(-4 + 2\cos\left((i-1)\pi/M\right) + 2\cos\left((j-1)\pi/N\right)\right)^2$ [2].
Initialize $v = (v_x, v_y) = 0 \in \mathbb{R}^{M \times N \times (P-1) \times 2}$.
while $\left\| v^{new} - v^{old} \right\| \geqslant TOL$ **do**

> % calculate displacement fields between slices
> **for** $k = 1, ..., P-1$ **do**
>> $F_x = 0;\ F_y = 0;$ % $\odot$ and $\oslash$: pointwise mult. and div.
>> **for** $s \in S$ **do**
>>> $\Delta I = I_{k+1} \circ \overleftarrow{p_k}(s) - I_k \circ \overrightarrow{p_k}(1-s);$
>>> $F_x = F_x + \Delta I \odot (\ s\, \partial_x I_k \circ \overrightarrow{p_k}(s) + (1-s)\, \partial_x I_{k+1} \circ \overleftarrow{p_k}(1-s)\ );$
>>> $F_y = F_y + \Delta I \odot (\ s\, \partial_y I_k \circ \overrightarrow{p_k}(s) + (1-s)\, \partial_y I_{k+1} \circ \overleftarrow{p_k}(1-s)\ );$
>> **end**
>> $v_{k_x}{}^{new} = \text{IDCT}\left(\text{DCT}\left(v_{k_x}{}^{old} - \tau F_x\right) \oslash D\right);$ % $v_{k_x}, v_{k_y} \in \mathbb{R}^{M \times N}$
>> $v_{k_y}{}^{new} = \text{IDCT}\left(\text{DCT}\left(v_{k_y}{}^{old} - \tau F_y\right) \oslash D\right);$
> **end**
> % calculate spline coefficients for object interpolations $\overleftarrow{p_k}, \overrightarrow{p_k}$
> Set up $d \in \mathbb{R}^{m \times n \times p \times 2}$ as in (3) with v^{new} and solve $A\,a = d$ with (4).

end
% calculate spline coefficients for intensity interpolation
Set up $d_I \in \mathbb{R}^{m \times n \times p}$ as in (6) and solve the systems $A\,a_I = d_I$ with (7).
% interpolate slices
$I_1{}^{\text{interp}} = I_1;\ l = 1;$
for $k = 1, ..., P-1$ **do**

> **for** $r = 1, ..., R-1$ **do**
>> $s = {}^r/R;$
>> % spline intensity interpolation of spline morphed slices
>> $\Delta I = I_{k+1} \circ \overleftarrow{p_k}(1-s) - I_k \circ \overrightarrow{p_k}(s);$
>> $I_l{}^{\text{interp}} = I_k \circ \overrightarrow{p_k}(s) + s\,\Delta I +$
>> $\quad + s\,(s-1)\,[s\,(h_k\, a_{I\,k+1} \circ \overleftarrow{p_k}(1-s) - \Delta I) + (s-1)(h_k\, a_{I\,k} \circ \overrightarrow{p_k}(s) - \Delta I)];$
>> $l = l + 1;$
> **end**
> $I_l{}^{\text{interp}} = I_{k+1};\ l = l + 1;$

end

L is invertible and only has one secondary diagonal on the first off-diagonal, and thus the spline coefficients a can be calculated by forward and backward substitution as follows:

$$\begin{cases} e_1 = d_1/L_{11} \\ e_k = (d_k - L_{k,k-1}\, d_{k-1})/L_{kk},\ k=2,...,P, \end{cases} \quad \begin{cases} a_P = e_P/L_{PP} \\ a_k = (e_k - L_{k,k+1}\, e_{k+1})/L_{kk},\ k=P-1,...,1. \end{cases} \quad (4)$$

For minimizing (2), we use gradient descent: alternatingly we calculate a new set of displacement fields through a descent step and calculate their spline interpolation – compare with the while loop of the pseudocode (Algorithm 1).

We could stop here and interpolate slices between the images I_k and I_{k+1} at any $z = z_k + s\,h_k$ by linearly combining the intensities of the warped images:

$$I^{\text{interp}} = (1 - s)\,I_k \circ \overrightarrow{p_k}(s) + s\,I_{k+1} \circ \overleftarrow{p_k}(1-s). \tag{5}$$

This would, however, result in kinks of the intensities along the trajectories and would result in a piecewise linear approximation.

We now construct a spline interpolation of the intensities along these trajectories. The correspondence interpolation is correct only locally along the interpolating axis, and registration errors between the corresponding points are summed up over several slices. Thus intensity information of slices further away should not have strong influence in the calculation of the interpolation. Because of the bounded supports $[z_k, z_{k+1}]$ of the piecewise interpolating polynomials p_k and the local dependencies between each other, encoded by the matrix A, we use the same approach of spline interpolation as before to smooth out the kinks of the intensities at the stitching positions. We compare the pure intensity differences at the stitching positions z_k and calculate the intensity spline coefficients a_I through solving the linear system $A\,a_I(\mathbf{x}) = d_I(\mathbf{x})$ with the following inhomogeneities:

$$d_{I1} = 3\left(\frac{I_2 \circ \overleftarrow{p_1}(1) - I_1}{h_1}\right), \quad d_{IP} = 3\left(\frac{I_P - I_{P-1}\circ\overrightarrow{p_{P-1}}(1)}{h_{P-1}}\right),$$
$$d_{Ik} = 3\left(\frac{I_k - I_{k-1}\circ\overrightarrow{p_{k-1}}(1)}{h_{k-1}} + \frac{I_{k+1}\circ\overleftarrow{p_k}(1) - I_k}{h_k}\right). \tag{6}$$

To make sure we can compare the images in (6) we added the registration evaluation points 0 and 1 to $\mathcal{S}$, recalling that Baghaie et al. [1] only registered them at $s = 1/2$. Preliminary experiments showed that forcing $I_k \circ \overrightarrow{p_k}(1/2)$ and $I_{k+1}\circ\overleftarrow{p_k}(1/2)$ to be similar does not guarantee that I_k and $I_{k+1}\circ\overleftarrow{p_k}(1)$ or $I_k\circ\overrightarrow{p_k}(1)$ and I_{k+1} are similar. The registration point $s = 1/2$ is still needed to optimize the third order polynomials. Other registration points can also be realized, in fact, every reslicing point could be used as a registration point. While solving $A\,a_I(\mathbf{x}) = d_I(\mathbf{x})$, we combine $d_{Ik}(\mathbf{x})$ at different locations z_k. In order to properly register them, we again utilize the tridiagonal structure of the matrix A: The lower triangular matrix L of the Cholesky decomposition $A = LL^T$ only has one secondary diagonal on the first off-diagonal. Therefore we can elegantly solve $L\,e = d_I$ and $L^T\,a_I = e$ with forward and backward substitution where for each subtraction the involved variables are warped to the mutual z-position:

$$\begin{cases} e_1 = d_{I1}/L_{11} & (k = 2,...,P) \\ e_k = (d_{Ik} - L_{k,k-1}\,(d_{Ik-1}\circ\overrightarrow{p_{k-1}}(1)))/L_{kk}, \end{cases} \begin{cases} a_{IP} = e_P/L_{PP} & (k = P-1,...,1) \\ a_{Ik} = (e_k - L_{k,k+1}\,(e_{k+1}\circ\overleftarrow{p_k}(1)))/L_{kk}. \end{cases} \tag{7}$$

Now we can interpolate slices between the images I_k and I_{k+1} at any $z = z_k + s\,h_k$, by replacing the linear combination (5) with (compare lower part of Algorithm 1)

$$\Delta I = I_{k+1} \circ \overleftarrow{p_k}(1-s) - I_k \circ \overrightarrow{p_k}(s)$$

$$I^{\text{interp}} = I_k \circ \overrightarrow{p_k}(s) + s\,\Delta I + s\,(s-1)\left[\,s\,(h_k\,a_{Ik+1} \circ \overleftarrow{p_k}(1-s) - \Delta I) + \right. \qquad (8)$$
$$\left. + (s-1)(h_k\,a_{Ik} \circ \overrightarrow{p_k}(s) - \Delta I)\right].$$

3   Experiments and Results

We implemented[1] the proposed algorithm in MATLAB. In all our experiments we linearly rescaled the images to values between 0 and 1, chose the parameters $\lambda = 10$ and $\tau = 10$ and stopped the optimization process when the mean square distance of the update is less than 0.1% for 10 consecutive iterations. For the in-slice image transformations ∘ we used bilinear interpolation during the registration phase and bicubic interpolation for (6)–(8). The optimization time of the proposed method is comparable to the time of the linear registration-based method. The complexity of one registration iteration is $\mathcal{O}(PMN\log(MN))$, where DCT with $\mathcal{O}(MN\log(MN))$ is the main contributor. Solving for the spline coefficients a with (4) is of order $\mathcal{O}(PMN)$.

The artificial scenario involves two tests: shape interpolation and intensity interpolation along the correspondence point trajectories. *Shape interpolation* involved non-linear, ellipsoidal movement of a 2D ellipse, see Fig. 2. We sampled 9 slices counterclockwise every eighth from 6 o'clock to 6 o'clock. Comparing the results of the proposed algorithm in the 2nd and the 3rd row in Fig. 2, we clearly see the benefit of the proposed against an intensity interpolation without calculating displacement fields. The second advantage of the proposed method is the non-linear movement estimation: In the 4th row we see the motion trajectory of the center points of the interpolated ellipses. The algorithm in [1] estimates the object motion piecewise linearly while the proposed approach calculates a spline interpolated motion field, which results in a better approximation of the true solution. In the 4th row on the right in Fig. 2 we clearly see the advantage of the proposed method with a leave-one-slice-out test. The calculated center point of the ellipse in the third slice is close to the analytic solution. To test the *intensity interpolation* we colored the ellipses along the slices with a sinusoidal, as shown in Fig. 2. The proposed method performs better than the proposed structure interpolation with only linear intensity (5) (spline reg).

For a second scenario, we use 42 datasets of the human spinal cord along the neck captured with a slicewise inversion recovery MR sequence (in-slice resolution 0.67 mm × 0.67 mm, slice distance 4 mm, slice thickness 8 mm) which we cropped for a centered view to a size of $120 \times 120 \times 10$ voxels; see Fig. 3. With a leave-one-slice-out interpolation we quantitatively evaluated how well the left out slices can be interpolated. In particular, we compared linear and cubic interpolation without registration, a reimplementation of the linear registration-based method of [1], the proposed interpolation with piecewise linear intensity

---

[1] https://mathworks.com/matlabcentral/fileexchange/63907.

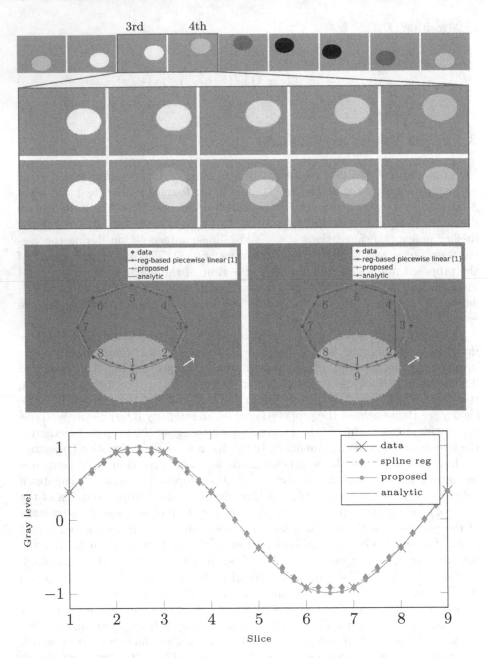

Fig. 2. *1st row:* 9 slices from left to right of a counterclockwise circling ellipse. *2nd row:* proposed interpolation between the 3rd and 4th slice. Images are shown in larger size than in row 1 for visualization without upsampling. *3rd row:* linear intensity interpolation. *4th row:* movement line of the center points of the interpolated ellipses of the proposed method compared against the slice interpolation of [1]. *4th row, right:* center points, when leaving the third slice out. *5th row:* gray values of the center points of the proposed solution are nicely interpolated compared to the analytic solution.

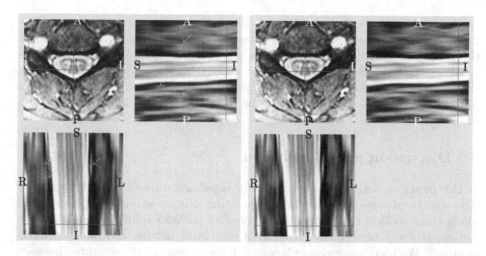

Fig. 3. Exemplary validation dataset. Slice interpolated with the method of Baghaie et al. [1] (*left*) and the proposed method (*right*). Upsampled and histogram equalized for better visualization. Transverse cut *(upper left)*, sagittal cut *(upper right)*, coronal cut *(below)*. In the sagittal and coronal cuts on the left kinks along the stitching positions are visible (yellow arrows). The proposed interpolation on the right is smooth. (Color figure online)

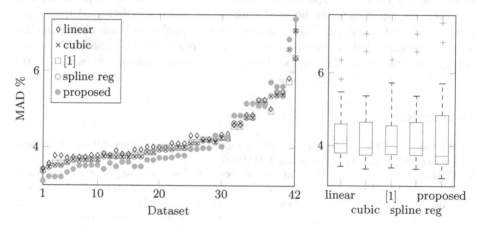

Fig. 4. Leave-one-slice-out interpolation of MR data. *Left:* MAD in percent of the interpolated slices compared to the corresponding left out slices of all datasets; datasets sorted for better visualization. *Right:* medians from left to right: 4.1, 3.9, 4.0, 3.9, 3.7.

changes (5) (spline reg), and the proposed method; see Fig. 4. As an evaluation metric we chose the mean absolute difference (MAD), comparing all the $(P-2)$ interpolated slices of the $(P-2)$ leave-one-slice-out interpolations to the left out slices of one dataset. In most datasets the registration process provided acceptable correspondences. In Fig. 4 we can see, that the proposed interpolation reaches a higher accuracy as long as the correspondences are accurate. The proposed method interpolated the datasets with 0.5% less error in intensity than [1]. Errors in the correspondences can increase the spline intensity interpolation error which also explains the slightly higher variance. Nevertheless, the proposed method improves on the slice interpolation capability of the pure intensity-based methods and of the registration-based linear interpolation methods.

4   Discussion and Conclusion

In this paper we derived a new method for registration-based slice interpolation. The structural motions along the interpolating axis are spline interpolated, and along these motion trajectories the intensities are also spline interpolated. We presented a way to solve the problem of combining motion and intensity interpolation. We used piecewise polynomial interpolators of degree three between the slices and the additional free degrees of freedom to even out the kinks at the stitching positions. The method produces two times differentiable structure- and intensity interpolations. Provided by accurate point correspondences between the slices, the smooth interpolation can be a better approximation than the ones from linear registration-based interpolations and from intensity-based cubic interpolations. To better guarantee point correspondences, we would like to point out that the proposed approach can be used with other, more sophisticated image distances and regularizations. The proposed slice interpolation framework is flexible and can be extended in several aspects. For example, the polynomial interpolators can be transformed to include bending of the interpolating axis, in case the slices are not parallel to each other.

References

1. Baghaie, A., Yu, Z.: An optimization method for slice interpolation of medical images [cs], February 2014. arXiv:1402.0936
2. Fischer, B., Modersitzki, J.: A unified approach to fast image registration and a new curvature based registration technique. Linear Algebra Appl. **380**, 107–124 (2004)
3. Frakes, D.H., Dasi, L.P., Pekkan, K., Kitajima, H.D., Sundareswaran, K., Yoganathan, A.P., Smith, M.J.T.: A new method for registration-based medical image interpolation. IEEE Trans. Med. Imaging **27**(3), 370–377 (2008)
4. Grevera, G.J., Udupa, J.K.: An objective comparison of 3-D image interpolation methods. IEEE Trans. Med. Imaging **17**(4), 642–652 (1998)
5. Hairer, E., Wanner, G.: Introduction à l'analyse numérique (2005) [Accessed: 28 July 2017]. http://www.unige.ch/~hairer/poly/poly.pdf
6. Leng, J., Xu, G., Zhang, Y.: Medical image interpolation based on multi-resolution registration. Comput. Math. Appl. **66**(1), 1–18 (2013)
7. Penney, G.P., Schnabel, J.A., Rueckert, D., Viergever, M.A., Niessen, W.J.: Registration-based interpolation. IEEE Trans. Med. Imaging **23**(7), 922–926 (2004)
8. Rueckert, D., Sonoda, L.I., Hayes, C., Hill, D.L., Leach, M.O., Hawkes, D.J.: Non-rigid registration using free-form deformations: application to breast MR images. IEEE Trans. Med. Imaging **18**(8), 712–721 (1999)

A Monte Carlo Framework for Low Dose CT Reconstruction Testing

Jonathan H. Mason[1(✉)], Willam H. Nailon[1,2], and Mike E. Davies[1]

[1] Institute for Digital Communications,
University of Edinburgh, Edinburgh EH9 3JL, UK
{j.mason,mike.davies}@ed.ac.uk
[2] Department of Oncology Physics, Western General Hospital,
Edinburgh Cancer Centre, Edinburgh EH4 2XU, UK
bill.nailon@luht.scot.nhs.uk

Abstract. We propose a framework using freely available tools for the synthesis of physically realistic CT measurements for low dose reconstruction development and validation, using a fully sampled Monte Carlo method. This allows the generation of test data that has artefacts such as photon starvation, beam-hardening and scatter, that are both physically realistic and not unfairly biased towards model-based iterative reconstruction (MBIR) algorithms. Using the open source Monte Carlo tool GATE and spectrum simulator SpekCalc, we describe how physical elements such as source, specimen and detector may be modelled, and demonstrate the construction of fan-beam and cone-beam CT systems. We then show how this data may be consolidated and used with image reconstruction tools. We give examples with a low dose polyenergetic source, and quantitatively analyse reconstructions against the numerical ground-truth for MBIR with simulated and 'inverse crime' data. The proposed framework offers a flexible and easily reproducible tool to aid MBIR development, and may reduce the gap between synthetic and clinical results.

Keywords: Computed tomography · Simulation · Synthesis · Iterative reconstruction · Low dose

1 Introduction

MBIR algorithms offer accurate CT imaging from a significantly lower dose than traditional FBP [1]. In general, they infer the underlying image by coupling an explicit statistical physical measurement model with spatial regularisation. By enforcing sparsity through appropriate regularisers, model-based iterative reconstruction (MBIR) may offer the ability to reconstruct even from an insufficient number of measurements with reduced projections or limited angle acquisitions [2,3], which bears strong resemblance to the field of compressed sensing (CS) [4,5].

© Springer International Publishing AG 2017
S.A. Tsaftaris et al. (Eds.): SASHIMI 2017, LNCS 10557, pp. 79–88, 2017.
DOI: 10.1007/978-3-319-68127-6_9

A limitation in the development and validation of such reconstruction methods however, is that one often has no ground truth from real measurements, and the scanners themselves will often have been carefully optimised for use with FBP [6]. Although one can easily generate synthetic measurements using the forward model used explicitly in the chosen MBIR from a numerical test image, this will be committing the so-called 'inverse crime' [7,8], which will unfairly bias the MBIR accuracy. Additionally, any deficits or artefacts from the model will be suppressed. Ideally, one would like a tool for generating highly realistic CT measurements from arbitrary specimen and systems, that would be repeatable and open for other researchers to easily validate proposed methods.

Several proprietary tools have been detailed to offer accurate synthesis of CT measurements such as [9,10], which use approximate physical modelling with Monte Carlo and smoothing to allow sufficiently many measurements for FBP, since the computational cost of fully sampled Monte Carlo would in this case be extremely high. Alternatively, the open software package GATE [11] allows simulation of X-ray measurement systems with full photon modelling, and allows implementation on parallel computing architectures and GPUs.

In this article, we will detail a framework using GATE to allow fully sampled Monte Carlo simulation of CT systems, for the specific use of MBIR development and validation. Although a relatively low flux of photons can be reasonably calculated with this complete modelling approach, due to its cost, this is ideal for evaluating reconstruction from highly noisy and limited measurements, but where the artefacts are physically realistic. We implement this using a large parallel computational cluster.

To form the complete data framework for MBIR testing, we use SpekCalc [12] to generate X-ray spectra, the Adult Reference Computational Phantom (ARC-Phantom) [13] as specimen data, Oracle Grid Engine scripting language for the computational implementation, the Michigan Image Reconstruction Toolbox (MIR-Toolbox) [14] for algorithm development, with attenuation database [15] for parameterisation and quantitative analysis.

We test the framework in Sect. 3 with examples of polyenergetic fan-beam CT and polyenergetic cone-beam CT (CBCT), where we compare against MBIR from 'inverse crime' data and FBP as a baseline.

2   Physically Modelling CT Systems

2.1   Discrete Measurement Model

CT scanners generate a set of discrete samples of X-ray intensity, which may be accurately expressed as [8]

$$y_i \sim \text{Poisson} \left\{ \int_{\boldsymbol{\xi}_i} b_i(\xi) \exp\left(- \int_{\boldsymbol{\ell}_i} \boldsymbol{\mu}(\ell, \xi) \, d\ell \right) d\xi + s_i(\boldsymbol{\mu}, \boldsymbol{b}) \right\} \text{ for } i = 1, ..., N_{\text{ray}},$$

(1)

where N_{ray} is the number of measurements in discrete vector $\boldsymbol{y} \in \mathbb{R}^{N_{\text{ray}}}$, $\boldsymbol{\xi}_i, \boldsymbol{\ell}_i$ are the energy spectrum and integral path, $\boldsymbol{b}, \boldsymbol{s}$ are vector fields of incident flux and scatter respectively, and μ is the spatially and spectrally varying linear attenuation coefficient of the specimen. In reality, there should also be an additive thermal noise from the electronics [8,16], and though we are not actively modelling this component of noise, it may be added to the data after synthesis.

Important features of (1) are that the measurements are spectrally blind, there is a mapping from continuous physical space to discrete measurement space, and the additive scatter component is non-linearly dependent on both μ and b. Due to these facts, unambiguously inferring μ from y is an ill-posed problem. In practice, one can instead invoke a simpler model such as [17]

$$y_i \sim \text{Poisson} \left\{ \sum_{j=1}^{N_\xi} b_i(\xi_j) \exp\left(-[\boldsymbol{\Phi}\boldsymbol{\mu}(\xi_j)]_i\right) + s_i \right\} \text{ for } i = 1, ..., N_{\text{ray}}, \quad (2)$$

where $b, s \in \mathbb{R}^{N_{\text{ray}}}$, $\xi \in \mathbb{R}^{N_\xi}$ and $\mu \in \mathbb{R}^{N_{\text{vox}}}$ are all discretised vectors, and N_ξ, N_{vox} are the number of energy bins and image voxels respectively. The matrix $\boldsymbol{\Phi} \in \mathbb{R}^{N_{\text{ray}} \times N_{\text{vox}}}$ is the 'system operator' describing the line-of-sight path through the specimen for each measurement.

To parameterise the polyenergetic attenuation in (2), a common approach is to model the specimen as a composition of few material classes, such as water and bone in [17]

$$\mu(\xi) = [\boldsymbol{f}_w(\rho)m_w(\xi) + (1 - \boldsymbol{f}_w(\rho))m_b(\xi)] \odot \rho, \quad (3)$$

where $\boldsymbol{f}_w(\cdot)$ is class indicator function of the water or air like materials, $m_w(\cdot), m_b(\cdot)$ are mass attenuation coefficients of water and bone, and $\rho \in \mathbb{R}^{N_{\text{vox}}}$ is the energy independent mass density. Reconstruction directly into density can then be done through

$$\hat{\rho} = \underset{\rho \geq 0}{\text{argmin}} \, \text{NLL}(\rho; y) + \Psi(\rho), \quad (4)$$

where $\text{NLL}(\cdot; \cdot)$ is the negative log-likelihood function of (2) with (3), and $\Psi(\cdot)$ is some regularisation function such as the total variation (TV).

MBIR solves (4) using an explicit model such as (2). Since in reality the measurements are better modelled with (1), it is valuable to use this to synthesise data instead of (2), to characterise deficits in the approximation and avoid committing the 'inverse crime'.

2.2   Modelling the Source and Detector

Modelling the source and detector can be considered as a characterisation of the incident flux given by b in (1). To characterise this, we note it may be decomposed as

$$b_i(\xi) = \mathcal{R}(\xi)p(\xi)n_i \text{ for } i = 1, ..., N_{\text{ray}}, \quad (5)$$

where $\mathcal{R}(\cdot)$ describes the energy dependent response of the detector, $p(\cdot)$ is the probability density function for generation of a photon of given energy, and n_i is the number of photons generated for a given ray.

To model the spectrum of a real diagnostic source, we assign an energy to each generated photon according to an appropriate probability density function. For this, we focus on spectra from a Tungsten anode with various tube potentials and including any beam filtering in the path to detector, for which we use SpekCalc [12]. For example, Fig. 1a shows a 120 kVp source with 4 mm Aluminium equivalent inherent filtration

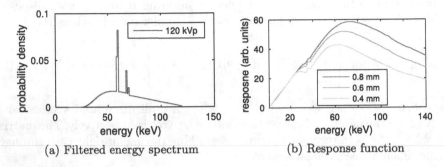

(a) Filtered energy spectrum   (b) Response function

Fig. 1. X-ray spectra for source and inherent filtration simulation and response function for CsI scintillator

Next is the spatial distribution of source flux as characterised by the vector $n \in \mathbb{R}^{N_{\text{ray}}}$ from (5). This represents a spatial probability density function, from which a given photon realisation is drawn. For this, we use distributions to replicate the effect of a bow-tie filters [18], which concentrate a higher flux into the centre of the specimen, reducing the radiation dose, the amount of scatter and beam hardening. In practice, to use these distributions in Monte Carlo simulation, we use a mirror image of the bow-tie distributions with a focal point at place halfway to the detector; variable intensity sources are natively supported in GATE. Although this approach gives a virtual point source, we note real sources will have a finite focal size [8]. Another deviation of this model from reality is that the variable thickness of the bow-tie will in practice induce a variation in spectrum, while in our modelling we currently use only a constant energy distribution for all rays.

Next, we will treat the modelling of an energy integrating detector, approximated by the response function $\mathcal{R}(\cdot)$ in (5), which is given ideally from the Beer–Lambert law as

$$\mathcal{R}(\xi) = \kappa \xi \left(1 - \exp \left(-\frac{\ell_d m_d^{\text{en}}(\xi)}{\rho_d} \right) \right), \tag{6}$$

where $m_d^{\text{en}}(\cdot)$ is the mass absorption coefficient of the scintillating material, ℓ is its thickness and ρ_d is its mass density. The scalar parameter κ in (6) is the constant converting an energy to a digital measurement, and will depend on the resolution of the analogue–to–digital converter of the sensor. Examples of the response functions for various thickness of Caesium–Iodine (CsI) with a density of $4.51\,\mathrm{g/cm}^3$ is shown in Fig. 1b and are quantified with arbitrary scaling of $\kappa = 1$. An important feature of modelling the response in this way is that the noise will be compound Poisson rather than exact Poisson in (2), which will be more representative of a real detector [8].

Finally, another common feature of the X-ray detector we would like to model is the scatter collimation grid [19], which consists of strips of lead parallel to the source beam to block scattered X-ray photons not travelling along the line-of-sight from the source. For the simulation of CBCT, we follow the specification of 'linear focused' grids from Soyee Product inc. (Seoul, South Korea), which are lead strips sandwiched between Aluminium. Our instance uses a grid ratio of 10:1, meaning the Aluminium spacers have dimensions of 2×0.2 mm; the lead strips have a dimension 2×0.05 mm. Unlike the source components we model as probability density functions, we physically build the scatter collimator by repeating, moving and rotating an a single collimation unit. For the modelling of fan-beam CT, we take the central slice of 2D grid we use for CBCT.

2.3   Specimen Material and Movement

The interaction of X-ray radiation with the specimen of interest is characterised with the attenuation coefficient $\mu(\xi)$ in (1) for a polyenergetic source. In order to model the interactions through Monte Carlo simulation, one requires the chemical composition and density of these materials, which in turn will characterise the attenuation. One such data set is the ACR-Phantom (ARCP) [13], of which a slice of the chest is shown in Fig. 2a, along with the pelvis in Fig. 2b. As we are concerned in this article with MBIR using the water–bone parameterisation in (3) [17], we will quantify the reconstructions in mass density. The mass-attenuation coefficients can be calculated from the appropriate compositions in the ACR-Phantom materials, and from the chemical attenuation database [15].

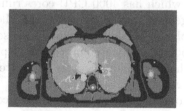
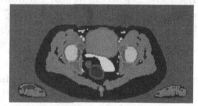

(a) Polyenegetic chest data   (b) Polyenegetic pelvis data

Fig. 2. Numerical specimens: (a) is a segmented material class map for polyenergetic simulation, with materials in arbitrary colours; (b) is the pelvis region (Color figure online)

The acquisition of CT data involves the revolution of source and detector around the specimen collecting projections. For simulation, we perform this process by instead rotating the specimen by discrete angles after a set number of photons. Examples of this along with an illustration of X-ray flight paths for 100 photons is illustrated in Figs. 3a and b.

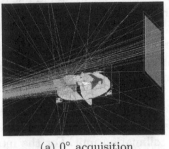
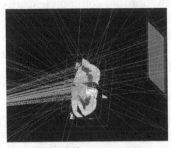

(a) 0° acquisition   (b) 100° acquisition

Fig. 3. Illustration of simulation of CBCT system for two different projection angles, for 100 photons (green) in each case (Color figure online)

It is from the position of the detector, and the movement of the specimen that will characterise the X-ray paths ℓ_i in (1). Since GATE will track photon interactions at a higher resolution that of the discrete ARC-Phantom, this will be only approximated by the 'system operator' Φ in the MIR-Toolbox [14], which will mitigate the 'inverse crime'.

2.4 Parallel Implementation and Data Consolidation

Since the interaction of each simulated photon is independent, the modelling of a complete CT acquisition may be run in a largely parallel manner. In our case, we utilised the Eddie cluster in Edinburgh, which has 4000 CPU cores running Oracle Grid Engine. We set up GATE to generate a file recording the photon intensity at discrete points on the detector plane, and split the simulation script into an appropriate number of indexed scripts, of number equal to a multiple of the number of projection angles. This can then be simultaneously submitted as an *array job* through Oracle Grid Engine scripting.

The output from the array job is therefore an indexed set of images corresponding to total detected energy. This is combined by summing images from the same projection angle in MATLAB. By replicating the system geometry of the GATE simulation with the MIR-Toolbox, these raw simulated measurements can then be reconstructed with MBIR with (4).

3 Examples and Testing

To illustrate the usage of the described data synthesis framework, we tested MBIR of fan-beam and CBCT geometries in low dose scenarios. In both cases, we evaluated the visual and quantitative accuracy of FBP and MBIR from Monte Carlo simulation, and inverse crime data generated directly according to (1).

In both cases reconstruction through MBIR is performed by solving the equation in (4) using (3) and (2), where we realised the operator $\boldsymbol{\Phi}$) using the MIR-Toolbox [14]. We used TV regularisation for $\mathcal{R}(\cdot)$ using the UNLocBOX [20], with parameters optimised for the root-mean-squared-error (RMSE) of mass density. Since to use (3) a segmentation of the water and bone classes is required, we provided each method with the hard bone structures.

3.1   Fan-Beam CT Example

In the first example, we tested a polyenergetic fan-beam CT system, using the ARC-Phantom chest data as shown in Fig. 2a. The geometry we use: 64.5 cm and 120 cm from source to object centre and source to detector respectively; a flat detector length of 85 cm with 512 equispaced elements; 90 equispaced projection angles distributed about 360°; a 120 kVp source with 4 mm Aluminium filtering as shown in Fig. 1a; a 0.6 mm CsI scintillator as shown in Fig. 1b; and a total of 1.5×10^9 photons. The synthesis took ~30 min with 90 parallel jobs on the Eddie cluster.

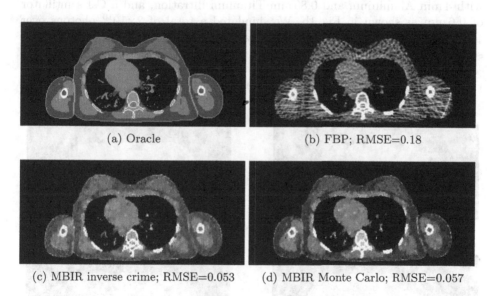

(a) Oracle   (b) FBP; RMSE=0.18

(c) MBIR inverse crime; RMSE=0.053   (d) MBIR Monte Carlo; RMSE=0.057

Fig. 4. Polyenergetic fan-beam CT reconstruction test with mass density grey-scale window [0.8,1.2]

Reconstructions from the polyenergetic fan-beam CT data are shown in Fig. 4. Key observations are significant streaking in the FBP as a result of photon starvation [18]. Between the Monte Carlo and inverse crime data, there is a visual difference in the soft tissue intensity and bone structure, where the latter appears closer to the ground truth. The intensity error of the simulated data can be explained by a deviation of materials such as soft bone and fat from the water–bone assumption [21]. Additionally, the inverse crime reconstruction has a 7% relative decrease in RMSE over data from our simulation framework. This is significant, as there are marked differences between using the very same method, which highlights that generating data from the model itself is overly optimistic in this case, and does not capture some of the shortcomings of the model using (3) with (2).

3.2 CBCT Example

The other example we will illustrate is the reconstruction of CBCT synthetic data. In this geometry, due to its wide field of view, there are large amounts of scatter that is often of the same order of magnitude as the measurements y [22]. In this case, the specimen is a 3D section around the pelvis of the ARC-Phantom [13]—a slice of this data is shown Fig. 2b.

For the acquisition, we set a geometry to match the 'half-fan' mode of Varian TrueBeam^{TM} system (Varian Medical Systems, Palo Alto CA, USA). For this, we used an offset detector, linearly focused scatter collimation grid, a 125 kVp source with 4 mm Aluminium and 0.89 mm Titanium filtration, and a CsI scintillator of 0.6 mm as shown in Fig. 1b. We simulated a total of 2×10^{10} photons over 160 projections, which is considerably less than around 900 as is typical for this scanner. Generating these measurements took ~3 h on the Eddie cluster.

We used fast adaptive scatter kernel superposition (fASKS) [19] to estimate the scatter. We also used this estimate to synthesise the data in the inverse

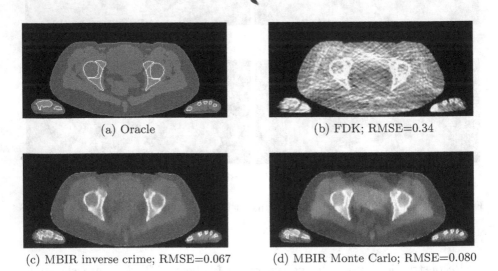

(a) Oracle   (b) FDK; RMSE=0.34

(c) MBIR inverse crime; RMSE=0.067   (d) MBIR Monte Carlo; RMSE=0.080

Fig. 5. Polyenergetic CBCT reconstruction test with mass density grey-scale window [0.6,1.4]; errors are calculated on full volume

crime case according to (2). For FBP, we used the fASKS estimate to correct the measurements.

Reconstructions in Fig. 5 show that the FBP again exhibits large amounts of streaking from the low dose. Even more so than the fan-beam case however, is the degree of difference between Monte Carlo and inverse crime data, which can be seen visually as shading in Fig. 5d and a 19% decrease in relative error. This highlights the importance of the dependency of real scatter as in (1), and motivates the use of more accuracy scatter estimation, which is suppressed with the inverse crime case.

4 Conclusions

We have introduced and tested a framework for synthesising CT measurements for MBIR development using freely available software. From our testing, we have shown it produces physically realistic reconstruction artefacts, such as intensity discrepancies or scatter shading that are not captured with inverse crime data. Future work will be in developing an easy to use interface for automating the scripting, data processing and consolidating, and make this freely available to enable easy replication. Additional physical effects such as finite focal size, detector lag [8], bow-tie shifting and variable spectra will also be investigated. We believe this work offers a transparent and valuable tool that should close the gap between numerical and real reconstruction results, and lower the barrier to clinical implementation of state-of-the-art methods.

Acknowledgements. This work was supported by the Maxwell Advanced Technology Fund, EPSRC DTP studentship funds and ERC project: C-SENSE (ERC-ADG-2015-694888). MD is also supported by a Royal Society Wolfson Research Merit Award.

References

1. Liu, L.: Reconstruction, model-based iterative: a promising algorithm for today's computed tomography imaging. J. Med. Imaging Radiat. Sci. **45**(2), 131–136 (2014)
2. Sidky, E.Y., Kao, C.M., Pan, X.: Accurate image reconstruction from few-views and limited-angle data in divergent-beam CT. J. X-ray. Sci. Technol. **14**(2), 1–30 (2006)
3. Hu, Z., Liang, D., Xia, D., Zheng, H.: Compressive sampling in computed tomography: method and application. Nucl. Instrum. Methods Phys. Res. Sect. A Accel. Spectrometers, Detect. Assoc. Equip. **748**, 26–32 (2014)
4. Candes, E.J., Romberg, J., Tao, T.: Robust uncertainty principles: exact signal reconstruction from highly incomplete frequency information. IEEE Trans. Inf. Theory **52**(2), 489–509 (2006)
5. Donoho, D.L.: Compressed sensing. IEEE Trans. Inf. Theory **52**, 1289–1306 (2006)
6. Pan, X., Sidky, E.Y., Vannier, M.: Why do commercial CT scanners still employ traditional, filtered back-projection for image reconstruction? Inverse Probl. **25**, 123009 (2009)

7. Kaipio, J., Somersalo, E.: Statistical inverse problems: discretization, model reduction and inverse crimes. J. Comput. Appl. Math. **198**(2), 493–504 (2007)
8. Nuyts, J., De Man, B., Fessler, J.A., Zbijewski, W., Beekman, F.J.: Modelling the physics in the iterative reconstruction for transmission computed tomography. Phys. Med. Biol. **58**(12), R63–R96 (2013)
9. De Man, B., Basu, S., Chandra, N., Dunham, B., Edic, P., Iatrou, M., McOlash, S., Sainath, P., Shaughnessy, C., Tower, B., Williams, E.: CatSim: a new computer assisted tomography simulation environment, p. 65102G, March 2007
10. Jia, X., Yan, H., Cerviño, L., Folkerts, M., Jiang, S.B.: A GPU tool for efficient, accurate, and realistic simulation of cone beam CT projections. Med. Phys. **39**(12), 7368–7378 (2012)
11. Jan, S., Benoit, D., Becheva, E., Carlier, T., Cassol, F., Descourt, P., Frisson, T., Grevillot, L., Guigues, L., Maigne, L., Morel, C., Perrot, Y., Rehfeld, N., Sarrut, D., Schaart, D.R., Stute, S., Pietrzyk, U., Visvikis, D., Zahra, N., Buvat, I.: GATE V6: a major enhancement of the GATE simulation platform enabling modelling of CT and radiotherapy. Phys. Med. Biol. **56**(4), 881–901 (2011)
12. Poludniowski, G., Landry, G., DeBlois, F., Evans, P.M., Verhaegen, F.: SpekCalc: a program to calculate photon spectra from tungsten anode X-ray tubes. Phys. Med. Biol. **54**(19), N433–N438 (2009)
13. ICRP Publication 110: Adult reference computational phantoms. Ann. ICRP **39**(2), 1 (2009)
14. Fessler, J.A.: Image Reconstruction Toolbox, 14 November 2014
15. Saloman, E.B., Hubbell, J.H., Scofield, J.H.: X-ray attenuation cross sections for energies 100 eV to 100 keV and elements Z = 1 to Z = 92. At. Data Nucl. Data Tables **38**(1), 1–196 (1988)
16. Chang, Z., Zhang, R., Thibault, J.-B., Sauer, K., Bouman, C.: Statistical X-ray computed tomography imaging from photon-starved measurements. SPIE Comput. Imaging **9020**, 90200G (2014)
17. Elbakri, I.A., Fessler, J.A.: Statistical image reconstruction for polyenergetic X-ray computed tomography. IEEE Trans. Med. Imaging **21**(2), 89–99 (2002)
18. Barrett, J.F., Keat, N.: Artifacts in CT: recognition and avoidance. RadioGraphics **24**(6), 1679–1691 (2004)
19. Sun, M., Star-Lack, J.M.: Improved scatter correction using adaptive scatter kernel superposition. Phys. Med. Biol. **55**(22), 6695–6720 (2010)
20. Perraudin, N., Kalofolias, V., Shuman, D., Vandergheynst, P.: UNLocBoX: A MATLAB convex optimization toolbox for proximal-splitting methods, February 2014
21. Schneider, U., Pedroni, E., Lomax, A.: The calibration of CT Hounsfield units for radiotherapy treatment planning. Phys. Med. Biol. **41**(1), 111–124 (1996)
22. Siewerdsen, J.H., Jaffray, D.A.: Cone-beam computed tomography with a flat-panel imager: magnitude and effects of x-ray scatter. Med. Phys. **28**(2), 220 (2001)

Multimodal Simulations in Live Cell Imaging

David Svoboda$^{(\boxtimes)}$ and Michal Kozubek

Faculty of Informatics, Masaryk University, Brno, Czech Republic
svoboda@fi.muni.cz

Abstract. During the last two decades a large amount of new simulation frameworks in the field of cell imaging has emerged. They were expected to serve as performance assessment tools for newly developed as well as for already existing cell segmentation or tracking algorithms. These simulators have typically been designed as single purpose tools. They generate the synthetic image data for one particular modality and one particular cell type. In this study, we introduce a novel multipurpose simulation framework, which produces the synthetic time-lapse image sequences of living endothelial cells for two different modalities: fluorescence and phase contrast microscopy, both in widefield or confocal mode. This may help in evaluating a wider range of desired image processing algorithms across multiple modalities.

Keywords: Cellular Potts model · Volumetric image data · Multimodal simulation · Cell imaging

1 Introduction

In the early 90s, the cell simulations represented rather a theoretical approach which was understood to be an important one but not practically used. Nowadays, namely due to the computational power and the capacity of contemporary computers, the development of new cell image analysis algorithms (e.g. segmentation, deconvolution) goes hand in hand with newly emerging cell simulation frameworks. The available simulation frameworks can generate the synthetic image data accompanied with absolute ground truth in large quantities. The simulated data are typically static [2,4]. Some research groups study the dynamic processes (tracking) and hence the availability of synthetic time-lapse image sequences [12] is required as well. However, even though many simulation frameworks emerged during the last years, they have been designed to be single-purpose. They typically generate just one cell phenotype and produce the images as if acquired with only one particular acquisition device. The design corresponds to the needs (running projects, available biological material) and equipment (available microscopes) of individual research groups that develop these tools. Most research groups are focused on the manipulation with data acquired using a fluorescence microscope [4,7,11]. The others handle bright field images [3,5], TIRF images [8], or SMLM images [9].

© Springer International Publishing AG 2017
S.A. Tsaftaris et al. (Eds.): SASHIMI 2017, LNCS 10557, pp. 89–98, 2017.
DOI: 10.1007/978-3-319-68127-6_10

To overcome the limitations of above-mentioned simulation frameworks, we designed a new simulation system that can generate the synthetic time-lapse image sequences depicting the living cell populations for two modalities: fluorescence and phase contrast microscopy. Such generated data are suitable for the evaluation of segmentation, tracking or registration task. The system is based on the modified cellular Potts model, that generates and manipulates with all the important data needed for further production of the synthetic image in both modalities. In particular, each cell is defined as a puzzle of subcellular components, each described with its refractive index [1] (needed for phase contrast simulation). Simultaneously, all the components are defined together with their internal structure [4], so that their virtual fluorescence staining is a straightforward process (needed for simulation of fluorescence microscopy). Finally, the generated synthetic images are submitted to a virtual optical system and virtual acquisition device to obtain the final image data. The description of fundamental parts of the simulation system follows in the next sections.

2   Methodology

The proposed simulation process consists of three principal phases [11]: generation of phantom, simulation of optical system, and simulation of acquisition electronic device. The first phase is fully controlled by the cellular Potts model (CPM). To allow different output for different modalities, the phantom, that is the output of this phase, is expected to be sufficiently complex. In this sense, we extended the standard Merks' CPM [6] into the 3rd dimension and made the cells content heterogeneous. In particular, the cell is now composed of three different components: nucleus, cytoplasm, and several mitochondria. In fact, Scianna and Preziosi [10] have already proposed an extension of CPM into the 3rd dimension and also introduced the subcellular components (they called them *compartments*). Nevertheless, their model did not guarantee the intra-cell compactness or inter-cell connectivity. Moreover, this model, even though very complex, could not distinguish the multiple occurrences of similar components in one cell. All of them were marked with the same identifier.

The aim of our modification is to provide a simple and straightforward 3D extension to a standard CPM and, in parallel, to overcome the imperfections of Scianna's CPM [10].

The basic as well as the modified version of our modified CPM is explained in the following subsection. The description of simulation of selected optical system and acquisition device is presented afterwards. The flowchart in Fig. 1 shows the workflow of the whole generation process.

2.1   Cellular Potts Model

Let $\Omega \subset \mathbb{R}^2$ be a two-dimensional lattice with each grid site $\mathbf{x} \in \Omega$ labeled with $\sigma(\mathbf{x}) \in \mathbb{N}_0$, called a spin. Note that the lattice with its sites and spins can be also understood as a discrete 2D image with individual pixels and pixel values. Each

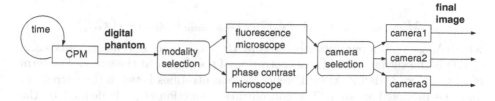

Fig. 1. Workflow of the simulation process.

studied object, e.g., cell, or embedding medium, consists of finite number of grid sites and possesses a unique spin. All sites belonging to a single object share the same unique spin number so that spin can be understood as a label of a given object in the lattice/image. By convention, the embedding medium, in which the real cells are immersed and which is commonly interpreted as a background, has spin number zero. One iteration of the CPM suggests to flip the spin of a randomly selected grid site $\mathbf{x}_s$ (source) to a spin $\sigma(\mathbf{x}_t)$ of a randomly selected neighbor $\mathbf{x}_t$ (target), and evaluates how this flip would affect the Hamiltonian H of the system:

$$\Delta H = \Delta H_{Adhesion} + \Delta H_{Shape} + \Delta H_{Chemotaxis}. \tag{1}$$

The term $H_{Adhesion}$ expresses the desire of individual grid site to either stay in contact with each other or to stay alone:

$$H_{Adhesion} = \sum_{\mathbf{x}\in\Omega, \mathbf{x}'\in N_x} \left(1 - \delta_{\sigma(\mathbf{x}),\sigma(\mathbf{x}')}\right) J_{\tau(\sigma(\mathbf{x})),\tau(\sigma(\mathbf{x}'))} \tag{2}$$

where $\delta_{x,y}$ is the Kronecker delta, $N_{\mathbf{x}}$ is a set of sites neighboring to $\mathbf{x}$, and $\tau(s)\colon \mathbb{N} \to \{\texttt{Medium}, \texttt{Cell}\}$ is a function associating each spin to a known type of object. A zero spin is associated with $\texttt{Medium}$ whereas all the positive values are mapped to $\texttt{Cell}$. Finally, the J's are cell-cell and cell-medium binding penalties.

The term H_{Shape} imposes geometrical constrains. In the simplest case, only the cell area (number of grid sites per cell) constraint is used:

$$H_{Shape} = \lambda_{shape} \overset{\text{number of cells}}{\sum_{\sigma=1}} (a_\sigma - A_{Cell})^2 \tag{3}$$

where λ_{shape} is a weight defining the influence of this term, a_σ is the current area of a cell with spin σ and A_{Cell} is an mean area each cell is expected to occupy in the lattice. The term $\Delta H_{Adhesion}$ (ΔH_{Shape}) expresses the difference between $H_{Adhesion}$ (H_{Shape}) calculated with the new suggested value of $\sigma(\mathbf{x}_s)$ and $H_{Adhesion}$ (H_{Shape}) with the original value.

Finally, the term $\Delta H_{Chemotaxis}$ expresses the cell ability to respond to the chemical stimulus. Each cell detects the concentration of signals (the biological material which is produced by each cell and which serves as an attractor to other cells) in its vicinity and tries to occupy the position with the highest positive gradient of concentration $c(\cdot, \cdot)$. The term is expressed as:

$$\Delta H_{Chemotaxis} = - \left(1 - \delta_{\sigma(\mathbf{x}_s),0}\right) \lambda_{chemical} \left[c(\mathbf{x}_t, t) - c(\mathbf{x}_s, t)\right] \tag{4}$$

where $\lambda_{chemical}$ is a parameter controlling the importance of cell chemotaxis and $c(\mathbf{x}, t)$ is the current (time t) concentration of the signals at the site $\mathbf{x}$. The term $c(\mathbf{x}_t, t) - c(\mathbf{x}_s, t)$ defines the difference in concentrations between the current $\mathbf{x}_s$ and the proposed $\mathbf{x}_t$ sites. The concentration function $c(\cdot, \cdot)$ is defined by the following equation (arguments were dropped):

$$\frac{\partial c}{\partial t} = D\nabla^2 c + \alpha(1 - \delta_{\sigma(\mathbf{x}),0}) - \frac{1}{\tau}\delta_{\sigma(\mathbf{x}),0}\, c \tag{5}$$

where α is the secretion rate constant of the signals released from the cells, τ is their half life in the medium, and D is the diffusion coefficient.

The probability of flipping the spin of the lattice site $\mathbf{x}_s$ to the spin $\sigma(\mathbf{x}_t)$ is then given as:

$$P\left(\sigma(\mathbf{x}_t) \leftarrow \sigma(\mathbf{x}_s)\right) = \begin{cases} e^{-\Delta H/T} & \text{if } \Delta H > 0, \\ 1 & \text{if } \Delta H \leq 0. \end{cases} \tag{6}$$

In the following text, we present the changes that we introduced to the standard CPM. In particular, these include the extension of standard CPM from 2D into 3D based on the fact, that $\Omega \subset \mathbb{R}^3$ is now a three-dimensional lattice, and the introduction of multi-component representation of each cell.

2.2 Subcellular Components

The standard CPM is composed of grid sites, each possessing a spin. This spin is understood as a label/index in the image. The set of grid sites with the same non-zero spin form a cell with a unique label. The grid sites with zero spin represent an embedding medium. In our model, each grid site $\mathbf{x} \in \Omega$ is again assigned a spin, which is newly defined as a triplet $\sigma : \mathbf{x} \to (Label, ID, Cell)$. Let us explain its individual elements in detail:

Label. This property defines the type of biological structure that the currently inspected grid site belongs to. In this study, we introduce the following set LABELS = {nucleus, cytoplasm, mitochondrion, medium, ECM}. Here, ECM stands for extra-cellular-matrix. The first three labels correspond to subcellular components. The last two labels define the non-cellular objects typically appearing in the specimens.

ID. Inside each cell, there may appear more than one mitochondrion. In order to distinguish between the individual occurrences of such objects and to avoid merging we introduce a unique identifier $ID \in \mathbb{N}_0$.

Cell. By using only the elements *Label* and *ID*, we are not able to recognize which grid site belongs to which cell. The component $Cell \in \mathbb{N}$ defines, which cell owns the currently inspected grid site.

With such a modified spin, we can easily perform the following operations over the grid:

- detect the interface between the individual cells,
- locate only the nuclei,
- remove the background

In accordance with the change of σ function, we also modify the τ function. Newly, the function τ is a projection of a spin $\sigma(\mathbf{x})$ into its first component, i.e.:

$$\tau(\sigma(\mathbf{x})) \rightarrow \tau((Label, ID, Cell)) \rightarrow Label \qquad (7)$$

The adhesion term $H_{Adhesion}$ is defined in the same way as in the standard CPM. The difference for the multicomponent model manifests itself in the number of adhesion $J_{.,.}$ terms [13]. Instead of $J_{cell,cell}$ and $J_{cell,medium}$ adhesion penalties we defined $J_{cytoplasm,ECM} = 3$, $J_{cytoplasm,medium} = 40$, $J_{cytoplasm,cytoplasm} = 3$, $J_{cytoplasm,nucleus} = 0$, $J_{cytoplasm,mitochondrion} = 0$. Note that the $J_{.,.}$ function is symmetrical. The unwanted connections (components should not touch each other) are set to a very high penalty, i.e. $J_{nucleus,ECM} = J_{nucleus,medium} = \infty$.

2.3 Sphericity of Components

Additionally to the standard CPM, where the geometrical term H_{Shape} is responsible for keeping the volume of all cells equal (see Eq. 3), we introduce the *sphericity*, which pushes the cells and some selected subcellular components (e.g. nuclei) to keep a roundish shape. The sphericity s_L of a component L is defined as:

$$s_L = \frac{\left(36\pi \text{volume}_L^2\right)^{\frac{1}{3}}}{\text{surface}_L} \qquad (8)$$

This newly defined property is very important, as without the additional restrictions the cells tend to arbitrarily prolongate and deflate. The volume and sphericity constraints are applied to each subcellular component individually:

$$H_{Shape} = \lambda_{volume} \sum_L \left(\frac{A_L - a_L}{a_L}\right)^2 + \lambda_{sphericity} \sum_L \left(\frac{S_L \ominus s_L}{s_L}\right)^2 \qquad (9)$$

where

$$x \ominus y = \begin{cases} 0, & y > x \\ x - y, & \text{otherwise} \end{cases} \qquad (10)$$

Here, the binary $\ominus$ operator realizes a subtraction with always positive result and S_L is an expected mean sphericity of components with label L. The operator $\ominus$ allows the components to be even more similar to sphere than required and still is not penalized. Further, $\lambda_{volume} = 1 \times 10^7$ and $\lambda_{sphericity} = 1 \times 10^8$ are weights defining the importance of volume and sphericity constrains, respectively. The zero value of $\lambda_{sphericity}$ means no restriction. Vice versa, the high values push the model to produce roundish shapes. We also normalize the deviations to avoid excessive changes of λ parameters caused when increasing/decreasing the lattice resolution. Note, that the normality requires very high value of λ parameters.

2.4 Modified Chemotaxis

The chemotaxis causes the cells in the scene to move and touch. This behaviour is controlled by the underlying field of concentration $c(\mathbf{x}, t)$ of signals. To push the cells, that are initially freely distributed in the medium, to attach the ECM, we changed the diffusion Eq. (5). We modified the Laplacian operator ∇^2 to control the direction of diffusion. The new operator $\nabla_{\mathbf{w}}^2$ is defined as follows:

$$
\begin{aligned}
\nabla_{\mathbf{w}}^2 f(x, y, z) = &-\left(\sum_{i=1}^{6} w_i\right) f(x, y, z) \\
&+ w_1 f(x, y, z-1) + w_2 f(x, y, z+1) + w_3 f(x, y-1, z) \\
&+ w_4 f(x, y+1, z) + w_5 f(x-1, y, z) + w_6 f(x+1, y, z)
\end{aligned}
\tag{11}
$$

where $\mathbf{w} = (w_1, w_2, \ldots, w_6)$ is a vector of weights that control the direction of diffusion of signals occurring in the medium. In this study, we used $\mathbf{w} = (0.8, 1.0, 1.0, 1.0, 1.0, 1.0)$. These settings cause the signals to be less diffused in upward direction. Due to chemotaxis, the cells less tend to grow in this direction. As a result they attach to the extracellular matrix which is located at the bottom of the specimen. This simply simulates the gravity force.

2.5 Connectivity

In order to keep each cell to be compact (intra-cell compactness) and to avoid splitting the two neighbouring cells that have already been connected (inter-cell connectivity), we adopted the graph based approach that tackles with the connectivity of 2D CPM [13]. In this sense, each cell is understood as a node in the non-oriented graph. Splitting the connection between two cells corresponds to an edge removal. Ripping the cell into multiple pieces corresponds to graph node replication. Both these events are controlled every time the spin flip is suggested. This way, we can prevent from any unwanted behavior of the cell population.

2.6 Simulation of Optical Microscope and Detector

The final phase of the simulation process consists of imitating the virtual microscope and virtual acquisition device.

Optical system. To simulate either the fluorescence or phase contrast microscope, we employed two different frameworks: virtual fluorescence microscope [11] and virtual phase contrast microscope [14]. To feed the frameworks, we utilized the complex digital phantoms produced by our modified CPM (see Fig. 1).

When using the virtual fluorescence microscope, the selection of one particular subcellular component corresponds to staining of the component with a real fluorescent dye. Moreover, staining different component with different dyes can produce typical pseudocolor multichannel images (see Fig. 2(b)).

Before we utilized the virtual phase contrast microscope, we defined the refractive indices for all the cellular as well as non-cellular structures occurring on the microscopic slide (water = 1.335, ECM = 1.3406, nucleus = 1.39, cytoplasm = 1.36, and mitochondrion = 1.4 [1]).

Image detection. First, the blurred image was affected by photon shot noise with Poisson distribution to imitate the ambiguity of photon detection by the camera sensor. Further, in order to get typical real-looking image, we employed one of virtual cameras, that are uniquely described by the resolution of their sensor, dark current signal and the Gaussian noise produced by amplifier.

3   Results and Discussion

The digital phantom generated using the proposed system (see Fig. 1) is a volumetric image, a 3D extension of standard representation of cellular Potts model. Unlike the common understanding of sigma value, which is a scalar, we redefine it as a triplet. Technically, this can be understood as a collection of three individual images (of the same size). The first stores the component labels, the second takes care of component identifiers, and the last one defines which cell the given component belongs to. Medium and extracellular matrix are examples of components that are not part of any cell.

The data stored in these three parallel fully 3D images are used to produce the final real-like looking synthetic images for the given pre-selected modality. An example of the third image, which records all the available cells in the specimen, is depicted in Fig. 2(a). The two possible outputs for two different modalities are shown in Fig. 2(b) and (c). The generated data are subsequently suitable for benchmarking of standard segmentation, tracking or registration tasks.

The reader should also keep in mind that the proposed framework is derived from the standard CPM, i.e., it straightforwardly adopts the ability to simulate the dynamic processes occurring in living cell populations. In particular, the parameters of the CPM framework control the willingness of cells to connect, to stay rounded or elongated, to attach to ECM, to have the membrane either smooth or jagged etc. As a result, the parameters influence the behaviour of the simulated population but due to the randomness of CPM framework, the different runs of the simulation with the same parameters produce different results. The values of the parameters, that were used for the generation of dozens of real-like looking cell populations (one sample image set is depicted in Fig. 2 and available from project web-pages[1]), are explained in the previous sections.

Regarding the plausibility of our generated data, we rely on the fact, that the introduced framework is a puzzle of several well-defined and already proved frameworks. The basic building block is a CPM [6,13] defining the proper shape and dynamics. Further, the texture of cell interior for fluorescence microscopy together with image acquisition is adopted from [11]. Analogously, the phase contrast-like looking images are produced by the model introduced in [14].

As we understand, that the model we proposed, cannot exactly meet the requirement of all the developers of cell segmentation/tracking/registration algorithms, we offer the source codes of our framework (see Footnote 1) for free such that any user can modify it to fit her/his needs. The code is completely written

---

[1] http://cbia.fi.muni.cz/projects/multicomponent-cpm.html.

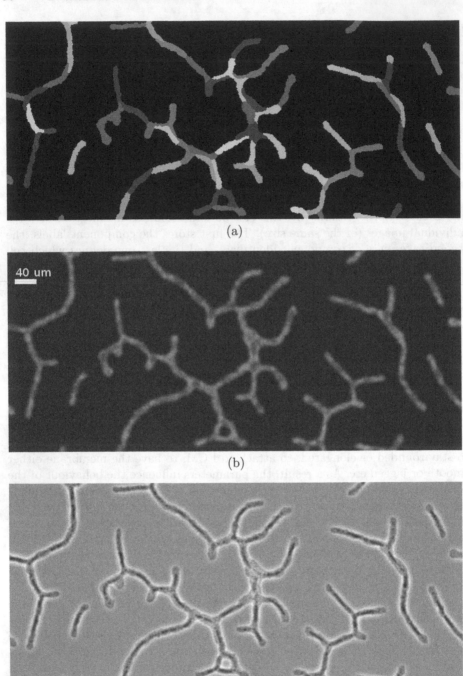

Fig. 2. An example of synthetic image data representing population of endothelial cells produced by the proposed simulation framework. From top to bottom: (a) Labeled digital phantom image with each cell bearing its unique label, (b) the output image imitating the acquisition with fluorescence microscope, where nucleus is depicted in red channel whereas the proteins, appearing in cytoplasm, are visualized in green channel, (c) the output image mimicking the phase contrast microscope. (Color figure online)

in C/C++ and works as a console application, i.e., without any limitation to operating system (tested under Linux Gentoo and MS Windows 10). We also accept the fact, that the CPM is commonly understood to be a rather slow simulation framework. For this purpose, we carefully optimized our codes to reduce the overall computation time. As a result, we were able to perform 3000 time steps over the scene consisting of $720 \times 720 \times 40$ voxels and containing 360 cells in $11\,h^2$.

4   Conclusion

In this study, we showed that the appropriate modification of cellular Potts model together with suitable virtual microscopes offer a powerful tool for simulation of microscopic image data for various modalities. In particular, we tested the suitability of this approach when generating the image data that resemble the real image data as if acquired using fluorescence or phase contrast microscope. The utilized approach is based on two main pillars:

Sufficiently complex model. As soon as the model is properly defined, we can generate a digital phantom suitable for particular modality. If someone plans to simulate the phase contrast microscope, for example, the refractive indices must be known for all the visible cellular parts. Moreover, to allow for the optical path length computation, which is an inevitable part of modeling of phase contrast microscope, the phantom must be defined fully in 3D. As for fluorescence microscopy, one has to tackle with the internal structure of visible cell parts. These are typically the chromatin (basic building block of nucleus) or some parts of cytoplasm visualized due to stained proteins.

Acquisition system modeling. In this study, we simulated the behavior of two types of microscopes. Due to sufficiently complex but still a simple model, we were able to produce the appropriate output for each of them. The simulation of fluorescence microscope is based on the on-line CytoPacq framework [11]. The phase contrast microscope is simulated using the model introduced and precisely described by Yin et al. [14].

In the future, the proper modeling of mitosis and apoptosis will be introduced to CPM to simulate to whole cell cycle. To make the system even more multipurpose, we also plan to support the differential interference contrast (DIC) microscopy and other modalities.

Acknowledgement. This work was supported by Czech Science Foundation, grant No. GA17-05048S.

---

[2] Reference computer: Intel(R) Xeon(R) QuadCore, 2.83 GHz, 32 GB RAM.

References

1. Dunn, A.K.: Light scattering properties of cells. Ph.D. thesis, University of Texas at Austin (1997)
2. Ghaye, J., Micheli, G., Carrara, S.: Simulated biological cells for receptor counting in fluorescence imaging. BioNanoSci. **2**, 94–103 (2012)
3. Korzynska, A., Iwanowski, M.: Artifical images for evaluation of segmentation results: bright field images of living cells. In: Piętka, E., Kawa, J. (eds.) ITIB 2012. LNCS, vol. 7339, pp. 445–455. Springer, Heidelberg (2012). doi:10.1007/978-3-642-31196-3_45
4. Lehmussola, A., Ruusuvuori, P., Selinummi, J., Huttunen, H., Yli-Harja, O.: Computational framework for simulating fluorescence microscope images with cell populations. IEEE TMI **26**(7), 1010–1016 (2007)
5. Malm, P., Brun, A., Bengtsson, E.: Papsynth: simulated bright-field images of cervical smears. In: International Symposium on Biomedical Imaging: From Nano to Macro, pp. 117–120. IEEE Press (2010)
6. Merks, R., Perryn, E.D., Shirinifard, A., Glazier, J.A.: Contact-inhibited chemotaxis in de novo and sprouting blood-vessel growth. PLoS Comput. Biol. **4**(9), e1000163 (2008)
7. Murphy, R.: CellOrganizer: image-derived models of subcellular organization and protein distribution. Methods Cell Biol. **110**, 179–193 (2012)
8. Rezatofighi, S.H., Pitkeathly, W.T.E., Gould, S., Hartley, R., Mele, K., Hughes, W.E., Burchfield, J.G.: A framework for generating realistic synthetic sequences of total internal reflection fluorescence microscopy images. In: International Symposium on Biomedical Imaging, pp. 157–160 (2013)
9. Sage, D., Kirshner, H., Pengo, T., Stuurman, N., Min, J., Manley, S., Unser, M.: Quantitative evaluation of software packages for single-molecule localization microscopy. Nature Methods-Tech. Life Scientists Chem. **12**(8), 717–724 (2015)
10. Scianna, M., Preziosi, L.: Multiscale developments of the cellular Potts model. Multiscale Model. Simul. **10**(2), 342+ (2012)
11. Svoboda, D., Kozubek, M., Stejskal, S.: Generation of digital phantoms of cell nuclei and simulation of image formation in 3D image cytometry. Cytometry Part A **75A**(6), 494–509 (2009)
12. Svoboda, D., Ulman, V.: MitoGen: a framework for generating 3D synthetic time-lapse sequences of cell populations in fluorescence microscopy. IEEE Trans. Med. Imaging **36**(1), 310–321 (2017)
13. Svoboda, D., Ulman, V., Kováč, P., Šalingová, B., Tesařová, L., Koutná, I.K., Matula, P.: Vascular network formation in silico using the extended cellular Potts model. In: IEEE International Conference on Image Processing, pp. 3180–3183, September 2016
14. Yin, Z., Li, K., Kanade, T., Chen, M.: Understanding the optics to aid microscopy image segmentation. In: Jiang, T., Navab, N., Pluim, J.P.W., Viergever, M.A. (eds.) MICCAI 2010. LNCS, vol. 6361, pp. 209–217. Springer, Heidelberg (2010). doi:10.1007/978-3-642-15705-9_26

Medical Image Processing and Numerical Simulation for Digital Hepatic Parenchymal Blood Flow

Marie-Ange Lebre[1], Khaled Arrouk[1], Anh-Khoa Võ Văn[1], Aurélie Leborgne[1],
Manuel Grand-Brochier[1], Pierre Beaurepaire[1], Antoine Vacavant[1(✉)],
Benoît Magnin[1,2], Armand Abergel[1,2], and Pascal Chabrot[1,2]

[1] Université Clermont Auvergne, SIGMA Clermont, CNRS,
Institut Pascal, 63000 Clermont-Ferrand, France
antoine.vacavant@uca.fr
[2] Centre Hospitalo-Universitaire,
63003 Clermont-Ferrand, France

Abstract. This paper deals with the personalized simulation of blood flow within the liver parenchyma, by considering a complete pipeline of medical image segmentation, organ volume reconstruction, and numerical simulation of blood diffusion. To do so, we employ model-based segmentation algorithms developed with ITK/VTK librairies, CATIA software for volumetric reconstructions based on NURBS and Abaqus solution for adapted simulation of Darcy's law. After presenting experimental results of each step, we explore scientific and technical bottlenecks so that a valid digital hepatic blood flow phantom may be developed in our future research, in direct relation with current open challenges in this domain.

Keywords: Medical image analysis · Model-based segmentation · Liver · Blood flow simulation · 3D reconstruction · NURBS

1 Introduction

The liver has multiple key biological functions and is a very complex organ, from both anatomical and physiological considerations [13], as suggested by Fig. 1: the shape of the liver can vary considerably from one patient to another; its vascular system is composed of two blood inflows (red and purple in Fig. 1 and one outflow (blue in Fig. 1), contrary to other organs like kidney, brain composed of one of each, moreover portal vein, hepatic artery and hepatic vein are respectively then subdivided into complex tree-like networks; in the liver, each hepatic cell (hepatocyte) has a connection to those networks (and bile duct, green in Fig. 1) by sinusoids and possesses many functions: synthesize proteins, detoxify, secrete bile, *etc.*

The very complex tree-like networks finish with capillaries, also called sinusoids (less than $10\,\mu$m), which are invisible on images acquired from medical

© Springer International Publishing AG 2017
S.A. Tsaftaris et al. (Eds.): SASHIMI 2017, LNCS 10557, pp. 99–108, 2017.
DOI: 10.1007/978-3-319-68127-6_11

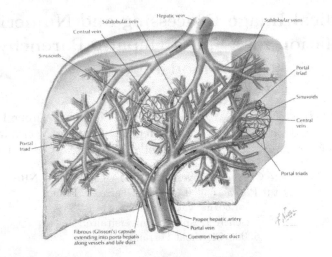

Fig. 1. Illustration of the complex vascular network of the liver with two input blood flows and one output. Image from [13] (Color figure online)

imaging systems such as MRI (Magnetic Resonance Imaging) or CT (Computed Tomography). Hence, simulating personalized blood transport and treatments (such as tumor embolization [12]) in an accurate way is a challenging question for the liver. Also, it would be a key to develop *in-silico* trials [21], to help medical doctors in defining embolization (transarterial chemo-embolization, radio-embolization, *etc.*) adapted to patients by using computer aided treatment planning, and to reduce animal experimentation for drug design and testing. The impact of such approach is high since liver cancer is the second leading cause of cancer-related death worldwide with 746,000 deaths in 2012 according to the World Health Organization (WHO) [22]. Therefore, numerous patients could benefit from these *in-silico* trials, by undergoing the best personalized treatments (as embolization) determined thanks to numerical testings.

In this paper, we present a complete pipeline devoted to simulate personalized blood flow within liver parenchyma (*i.e.* liver volume except vessels, thus comporting hepatic lobules). We also point out key scientific and technical problems of this process, and possible ways to solve them in future works. Another objective of this work is to draw the possible relations between image-based simulation and (model-based) medical image processing. The paper follows our pipeline and is organized as follows. Section 2 deals with the segmentation of liver volume and internal vessels, from CT and MRI volumes. Then, in Sect. 3, we explain how to obtain a valid 3D model appropriate for the simulation, which is exposed in Sect. 4. We finish by discussing this study and possible future works in Sect. 5.

2   Liver Segmentation in CT and MRI Modalities

Liver segmentation in MRI and CT is a challenging problem due to noise, low contrast and similar intensities with adjacent organs and tissues. Automatic liver segmentation is often performed in CT [3] but MRI provides more information for diagnosis purposes [1]. We have developed an automatic model-based method for both modalities. To do so, we first extract four statistical models with 68 livers segmented by clinical experts obtained from Shape2015 [10], IRCAD [14] and SLIVER07 [8] databases. The four models are constructed according to their variabilities (small to large) from a standard shape liver (mean dimensions of all volumes available in the datasets). Statistical model and all patient volumes have the same dimensions (voxel size: $1 \times 1 \times 1\,\mathrm{mm}^3$).

We first localize the liver on the images with the mean dimensions of a standard liver. This localization of the liver allows us to compute a threshold to isolate pixels that belong to the liver. After the thresholding on each slice, we apply a contour enhancement process. At this step we use the model the liver) as a probability map to localize the liver and we then perform an active contour segmentation method (fast marching) resulting in a binary mask. Finally, to erase errors due to over-segmentation by a process considering the global shape of the liver. Figure 2 illustrates results of the different steps.

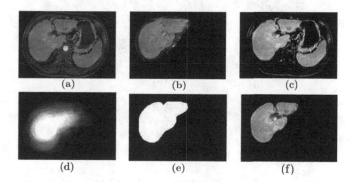

Fig. 2. Results of different step on MR images: (a) patient slice P_j with $j \in \{1,p\}$, (b) largest surface of the liver (threshold computation), (c) thresholding and contour enhancement, (d) liver model for localization and active contour method, (e) mask obtained, (f) segmentation result

In the second step, we extract the liver vessels within the 3D segmentation obtained previously from CT and MRI volumes. The contrast of the blood vessels in our images is quit good as a contrast agent injection is generally performed during the medical exam. Thus, we first tried a simple thresholding to segment the vascular network (see results in Fig. 3). Nonetheless, we also tried to apply two different vessel filters: the Sato vesselness based on the analysis of the Hessian matrix, which plays a role in a discriminating shape and orientation of tubular structures [16]; and the RORPO filter (Ranking the Orientation

Responses of Path Operators) [11], based on the notion of path operators from mathematical morphology. It allows a discrete, non linear and non local, 3D curvilinear structure analysis.

The automatic liver segmentation has been tested with 20 CT from the IRCAD database, 20 CT from the SLIVER07 challenge and 39 MR images from our radiology department. The ground truth of the liver segmentation is available for the SLIVER07 and IRCAD databases only, which permits us to calculate the mean Dice of our method, which is equal to $90,5\%$. The vessels extraction is tested on CT of the IRCAD database and MR images. Manual expert segmentations of the portal vein, the arterial vein and the venous system are available for the IRCAD database. The mean Dice is equivalent for the three vessels extraction methods, around 30%. The parameters are not yet optimized and more tests are needed, specially on MRI, but results are promising: Sato-filter is stable according to the different modalities but contains lot of noise, RORPO is promising for CT and results obtained with simple thresholding highly depend on patient's data. The entire process allows a 3D visualization of the patient liver with its vascular network, Fig. 3 illustrates results for two CT and one MRI volume.

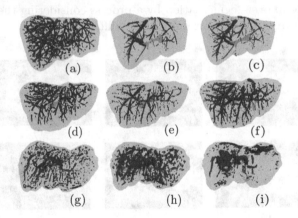

Fig. 3. Visualization of the liver segmentation (in light blue) and its vascular network (in dark blue). First two lines correspond to two CT and the third line corresponds to one MRI. Then (a), (d), (g) represent results with Sato filter, (b), (e), (h) results with the RORPO algorithm and (c), (f), (i) are calculated with a simple thresholding process (Color figure online)

3   Liver Components Reconstruction

In this work, the analysis is performed using a finite element (FE) solver. FE solver uses the geometric information provided by the 3D Computer-Aided Design (CAD) models. These 3D models can be a solid model or a surface model such as Non-Uniform Rational Basis Spline (NURBS, see *e.g.* [15]). Such models are not directly obtained from the CT, and therefore the NURBS model needs to be reconstructed in order to maintain the workflow required by the FE solver.

3.1 Liver Reconstruction

From the liver obtained by segmenting medical images (Sect. 2), we obtain a 3D triangular mesh by using the marching cubes algorithm, meaning that 3D points are spaced wrt. the segmented image resolution (*i.e.* the voxel size is $1 \times 1 \times 1\,\text{mm}^3$). We also use a Laplacian smoothing operator to enhance the 3D mesh. To produce this mesh, we employ the Visualization Toolkit VTK, and export the reconstructed liver in the STL format (Stereolithography), as shown in Fig. 4a. We import the mesh into the CAD software CATIA®, which can be used to convert the 3D surface polygonal mesh into a NURBS surface model, as shown in Fig. 4b. This closed surface is subsequently filled to obtain a solid model needed to perform the FE analysis.

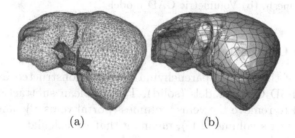

(a)   (b)

Fig. 4. Reconstruction of the liver model: (a) Original surface mesh. (b) Volumetric CAD model. From an IRCAD sample [14]

3.2 Venous System Reconstruction

The model of the venous system is reconstructed from a surface polygonal triangular mesh (see Fig. 5a), but the procedure used for the liver cannot be directly applied. In fact, the preparation of a FE model for veins from a 3D CAD model is a difficult task, because the geometry of the veins is more complex, which may lead to distorted or non physical NURBS. The 3D surface model of the veins contains a large number of faces, some of which may be narrow or feature short edges that are smaller than the required FE size for 3D mesh generation. In our case, for instance, we frequently observed intersections between the opposite walls of a vein or NURBS with excessive curvature radii, which cannot be meshed by the FE software. Therefore, the radii of the veins have been slightly increased between 1–1.5 mm, in an adaptive way considering the mesh geometry by means of CATIA. The reconstructed and modified CAD model of the veins is shown in Fig. 5b. The hepatic artery is not included in this model, as it is considerably smaller than the vena cava and the hepatic vein, the input model used here did not include sufficient information.

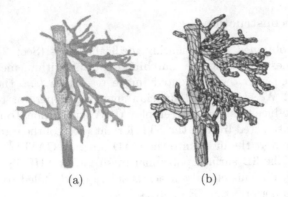

(a)   (b)

Fig. 5. Construction of the geometric vein model from an IRCAD example [14]: (a) Original surface mesh. (b) Volumetric CAD model

3.3   Boolean Operations

The geometry of the hepatic parenchyma HP is reconstructed from the previously described 3D CAD models (solid). Two Boolean subtractions are subsequently applied to remove the veins' volumes (portal veins PV and hepatic vein HV) from the liver's volume (LV), meaning that we calculate:

$$HP = (LV \setminus PV) \setminus HV. \tag{1}$$

An assembly model including all the reconstructed solids is prepared as shown in Fig. 6.

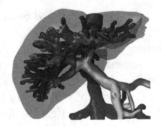

Fig. 6. Geometric model of the liver with the modified venous system   (IRCAD sample [14])

4   Numerical Simulation of Blood Transport Within Liver Parenchyma

A porous medium model of the liver is developed in this paper. A similar approach at the microscopic scale is described in the literature [2,19]. The simulations are focused on the hepatic parenchyma and a 3-dimensional volume model is implemented. Simulation of the flow of blood is possible using computational fluid dynamics (see *e.g.* [18, 20]) but this approach is not considered here. The larger veins and arteries can be explicitly identified from the CT. They are subsequently excluded from the analysis and it is assumed that they can be replaced by appropriate boundary conditions. The smaller veins cannot be identified from the CT, as there are smaller than the resolution of the images. It is assumed as a simplifying hypothesis that all the unidentified veins and arteries behave as the parenchyma, and they are modeled with the properties of the porous medium.

4.1 Constitutive Equations

Darcy's law is used to model the flow of blood in the hepatic parenchyma; it is expressed as:

$$\mathbf{q} = \frac{k}{\mu} \nabla P, \tag{2}$$

where $\mathbf{q}$ denotes the flux of the fluid (expressed in volume of fluid per unit of surface and per unit of time, *i.e.* in m/s), ∇P denotes the gradient of the pressure of the fluid within the pores (liver lobules), k and μ are respectively the permeability of the bulk material and the viscosity of the fluid. The influence of gravity is neglected in Eq. 2, as we assumed that the difference of pressure in the portal vein and in the hepatic vein causes the blood flow; and that the volumetric forces have second order effects. The second constitutive equation is the conservation of the mass:

$$\nabla \cdot \mathbf{q} = 0, \tag{3}$$

where $\nabla \cdot$ is the divergence operator. It should be noted that the flux is not the actual velocity of the fluid, as it travels only in the pores and the solid material reduces the available space.

Equations 2 and 3 do not include any partial derivative of the fluid flux and pressure with respect to time as they describe the flow within the porous medium in steady state condition. This approximation allows us to reduce the numerical efforts associated with the analysis, and has been applied with success in the literature (see *e.g.* [2, 19]). Homogeneous isotropic material properties are used for the hepatic parenchymal material, we have set $k = 1.56 \cdot 10^{-14} \, m^2$ and the blood viscosity $\mu = 0.0024 \, Pa.s$.

The method is implemented in the commercial FE solver Abaqus. Darcy's law is available in this software, which is used by civil engineers to solve soil mechanics and hydraulics problems. 4-node tetrahedral elements are used, as they are versatile elements suitable for complex geometries. The model includes 585,219 elements and 110,266 nodes in total.

4.2 Boundary Conditions

The first boundary condition consists of applying no blood flux at the wall of the vein, nor at the surface of the liver, which is expressed as:

$$\mathbf{q} \cdot \mathbf{n} = 0 \tag{4}$$

at any point of a surface where this flux boundary condition is prescribed, n being the normal vector of the surface. This is the default boundary condition applied by the solver for all the free surfaces, excepted if another boundary condition is explicitly applied.

Specific boundary conditions are applied at the ends of the veins as they apply in the geometry reconstructed from the medical image. These veins are not included in the FE model, and their end surfaces are modeled as an inlet or as an outlet. Two modeling strategies are applicable; they consist of applying: (i) the fluid flux; (ii) the pressure of the fluid on the pores. The second strategy is used here as relevant information on the pressure in the hepatic and portal vein is available in the literature [19]. The pressure is 587 Pa at the ends of the portal veins and 200 Pa at the ends of the hepatic vein.

4.3 Experimental Results

Figure 7 shows the results of the FE analysis, the fluid pressure and flux are determined. It is observed that both quantities exhibit higher values in the vicinity of the veins end (as they are observed from the medical images).

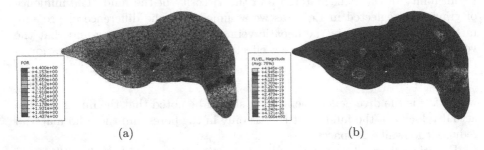

(a)   (b)

Fig. 7. Results of the FE analysis (a) Fluid pressure in the parenchyma. (b) Blood flux

5 Discussion

In this paper, we have presented a complete pipeline dedicated to the simulation of blood flow within liver parenchyma from personal medical image data. We now propose to consider different technical and scientific issues, and possible solutions to be developed as future works.

Simulation outcome validation. As presented in Fig. 7, numerical simulation based on Darcy's law enables the computation of blood flow within liver parenchyma, by calculating flow pressure or velocity in each FE node of the 3D reconstructed object. To validate this process, we have to take into account the blood flow coming from liver vessels, by incorporating fluid dynamics. In this case, flow should be synchronized with cardiac rhythm, with the support of ECG signal for instance. To validate our digital blood flow, we could study the correlation with blood flow estimation from several image modalities (ultra-sound imaging, MR angiography, *etc.*) [4].

CT or other modalities only offer a coarse representation of liver vessels. A solution could be to reconstruct finer vessels by heuristics based on geometrical and anatomical features upon vascular shapes in this organ, as proposed by [17]. In Fig. 7, we can observe some parts of the liver with an abnormal flux and/or pressure (see left-most and bottom-right parts in particular) wrt. the rest of the organ. In reality, liver vascular network is organized so that every hepatic lobules participate in the treatment of blood. As a consequence, the vessels we have employed from IRCAD segmentation in this study do not have a sufficient precision to accomplish this task.

Also, simulation should also be driven by a multi-scale approach, so that we consider blood flow dynamics within hepatic lobules, like in [19]. This means that we should be able to draw the relation between possibly cirrhotic liver reconstructed from macroscopic images (CT, MRI) and microscopic data (histology).

Image processing quality and robustness. In our study, liver extraction method achieve an accuracy (Dice measure) of approximately 30% wrt. manual annotation provided by IRCAD dataset (see Fig. 3). And visual appreciation of results from MRI data suggest that the quality of vascular reconstruction would be even worst. From previous observations, we may suppose that simulation based on such reconstructions will suffer from a lower outcome quality compared to the one we have obtained with IRCAD segmentations in this paper. However, we have to be aware that image-based quality measurement is not forced to be correlated to simulation performance measurement. And if we consider *in-silico* trial as the final goal of our work, digital blood flow assessment should be the best way to judge the quality of previous segmentation tasks. This is also related to the current concern about evaluating the reproducibility and robustness of image processing tasks, by considering more applications [9].

Scalability, benchmarking and big data. In our pipeline, several operations have been produced by supervised manipulations: liver and vascular reconstruction, as exposed in Figs. 4 and 6 in CATIA, input/output labeling of vessels in Abaqus, *etc.* To be able to handle a large number of images (as our dataset of 39 MRI volumes, and even larger patient cohorts), automatic procedures should be developed. In this case, a first solution is to design home-made algorithms or use open-source solutions for volume reconstruction [6] and blood flow simulation [7]. Producing such automatic processes will also help in validating image processing tasks and the possible underlying models or atlases (as we propose in this article for the liver) for large amounts of data.

References

1. Bereciartua, A., et al.: Automatic 3D model-based method for liver segmentation in MRI based on active contours and total variation minimization. Biomed. Signal Process. Control **20**, 71–77 (2015)
2. Bonfiglio, A., et al.: Mathematical modeling of the circulation in the liver lobule. J. Biomech. Eng. **132**(11), 1–10 (2010)

3. Campadelli, P., et al.: Liver segmentation from computed tomography scans: a survey and a new algorithm. Artif. Intell. Med. **45**, 185–196 (2009)
4. Chow, P.K., et al.: The measurement of liver blood flow: a review of experimental and clinical methods. J. Surg. Res. **112**(1), 1–11 (2003)
5. El-Serag, H.B.: Hepatocellular carcinoma. New Engl. J. Med. **365**, 1118–1127 (2011)
6. Hang, S.: TetGen, a delaunay-based quality tetrahedral mesh generator. ACM Trans. Math. Softw. **41**(2), 11 (2015)
7. Hecht, F.: New development in FreeFem++. J. Numer. Math. **20**(3–4), 251–265 (2012)
8. Heimann, T., et al.: Comparison and evaluation of methods for liver segmentation from CT datasets. IEEE Trans. Med. Imaging **28**(8), 1251–1265 (2009)
9. Kerautret, B., Colom, M., Monasse, P. (eds.): RRPR 2016. LNCS, vol. 10214. Springer, Cham (2017)
10. Kistler, M., et al.: The virtual skeleton database: an open access repository for biomedical research and collaboration. J. Med. Internet Res. **15**(11), e245 (2013)
11. Merveille, O., et al.: Curvilinear structure analysis by ranking the orientation responses of path operators. IEEE Trans. Pattern Anal. Mach. Intell. **1** (2017). doi:10.1109/TPAMI.2017.2672972
12. Rammohan, E., et al.: Embolization of liver tumors: past, present and future. J. Radiol. **4**(9), 405–412 (2012)
13. Netter, F.H.: Atlas of Human Anatomy. Saunders, Philadelphia (2014)
14. Research Institute against Digestive Cancer. IRCAD dataset. http://www.ircad.fr/research/3d-ircadb-01/
15. Rogers, D.F.: An Introduction to NURBS. Morgan Kaufmann, San Francisco (2001)
16. Sato, Y., Nakajima, S., Atsumi, H., Koller, T., Gerig, G., Yoshida, S., Kikinis, R.: 3D multi-scale line filter for segmentation and visualization of curvilinear structures in medical images. In: Troccaz, J., Grimson, E., Mösges, R. (eds.) CVRMed/MRCAS -1997. LNCS, vol. 1205, pp. 213–222. Springer, Heidelberg (1997). doi:10.1007/BFb0029240
17. Schwen, L.O., Preusser, T.: Analysis and algorithmic generation of hepatic vascular systems. Int. J. Hepatol. **2012**, Article ID 357687 (2012)
18. Schwen, L.O., et al.: Spatio-temporal simulation of first pass drug perfusion in the liver. PLoS Comput. Biol. **10**(3), e1003499 (2014)
19. Siggers, J.H., et al.: Mathematical model of blood and interstitial flow and lymph production in the liver. Biomech. Model. Mechanobiol. **13**(2), 363–378 (2014)
20. Sousa, L.S., et al.: Finite element simulation of blood flow in a carotid artery bifurcation. In: Congress on Numerical Methods in Engineering, Coimbra (2011)
21. Viceconti, M., et al.: In silico clinical trials: how computer simulation will transform the biomedical industry. Avicenna-ISCT, Avicenna Project (2016)
22. World Health Organization: Liver cancer. Estimated incidence, mortality, prevalence worldwide in 2012. http://globocan.iarc.fr/old/FactSheets/cancers/liver-new.asp

Author Index

Printed in the United States
by Bookmaster

Printed in the United States
By Bookmasters